# GOOD INTENTIONS IN GLOBAL HEALTH

## ANTHROPOLOGIES OF AMERICAN MEDICINE: CULTURE, POWER, AND PRACTICE

General Editors: Paul Brodwin, Michele Rivkin-Fish, and Susan Shaw

# Good Intentions in Global Health

*Medical Missions, Emotion, and*
*Health Care across Borders*

Nicole S. Berry

NEW YORK UNIVERSITY PRESS
New York

NEW YORK UNIVERSITY PRESS
New York
www.nyupress.org

© 2024 by New York University
All rights reserved

Please contact the Library of Congress for Cataloging-in-Publication data.

ISBN: 9781479825363 (hardback)
ISBN: 9781479825370 (paperback)
ISBN: 9781479825424 (library ebook)
ISBN: 9781479825400 (consumer ebook)

This book is printed on acid-free paper, and its binding materials are chosen for strength and durability. We strive to use environmentally responsible suppliers and materials to the greatest extent possible in publishing our books.

Manufactured in the United States of America

10 9 8 7 6 5 4 3 2 1

Also available as an ebook

*To Noelle,*

*for making it possible*

*for me to write this book*

CONTENTS

# PROLOGUE

This is a book about contemporary global health, prompted by the exploration of an increasingly popular phenomenon—a particular form of clinically engaged travel that I refer to as a "short-term medical mission" (STMM).[1] This book stems from a specific fieldwork event that brought short-term medical missions to the forefront of my thinking. While I had previously considered STMMs peripheral to my research, this experience highlighted them as a phenomenon meriting sustained ethnographic attention. Perhaps, more importantly, this seed story demonstrates how my entanglement with STMMs has fundamentally altered the ways in which I think about the practices and actions in the domain referred to as "global health."

One morning in 2002, I interviewed Luz, a Kaqchikel Maya woman a few years older than I was, and this was the conversation that inevitably led to my research on STMMs. I met her during the second year of fieldwork for my dissertation, which explored global initiatives to decrease maternal mortality. I was sitting in the courtyard of her family's compound in Sololá, Guatemala, interviewing her about her childbearing experiences and the complications that might have ensued. Luz was the second woman I met who was suffering from a prolapsed uterus—a condition in which the uterus slips out of the vaginal opening. She described in detail what this meant to her everyday life. For example, she would routinely walk into the countryside to gather firewood for cooking. She would tie the firewood together into a large bundle and then use ropes to attach that bundle to a headband. To bring the firewood home, she would squat down, position the bundle on her back, put the headband on her forehead, and then push up to standing under the weight. As a result of this exertion, her uterus would inevitably fall out between her legs, and she would have to endure the wetness and the discomfort of the flesh scraping against her thighs all the way home. What could she do? she asked me. If she put the wood down to push her uterus back inside her body, it would just fall out again when she picked up the wood. Luz's suffering increased as her uterus fell out more routinely. Moreover, she told me, she was still getting pregnant despite her weak uterus. On that day, Luz made me promise to tell her if I ever found a way to help her.

The academic ethics board regulating human subject research allowed me to exchange a bar of soap for Luz's life story. As Cal Biruk (2018:101) details in their ethnography *Cooking Data*, such exchanges are enfranchised within a research ethics framework that imagined "an ideal-type agentive subject who participates altruistically in research."[2] Not surprisingly, the ethical standards on which my participants insisted were quite different. When I entreated them to tell me about their lives and opinions, they viewed my interest as the first move in an ongoing relationship of exchanges. Like many other people I interviewed, Luz leveraged our relationship, in this case by asking me to help her to seek medical care.

Months after Luz's interview, I was buying groceries in a nearby town when I saw a flier advertising a *jornada* (the local name for a medical mission) of doctors coming from Toronto, Canada, to perform surgeries in Sololá on local people in need.[3] Taped to a telephone pole, the announcement listed the specific types of problems that could be addressed, gynecological issues among them. Thinking of Luz, I ripped off a little fringe slip from the bottom of the flier with the time and place where the surgeons would evaluate potential patients. Later that day, I walked to Luz's house to talk to her about the jornada. Her family had many questions; for instance, Who were the doctors? Why were they coming to Guatemala and doing these surgeries? How did I know that they would be able to treat Luz? Where and when would they perform the surgeries? How much would it cost? I could not answer any of these questions. But I told them I would be happy to accompany Luz to the evaluation to see if surgery was an option for her and to ask our questions. Little did I know that tearing this slip of paper off the advertisement would be a fateful decision, setting in motion a chain of events that would lead to this book.

On the morning of the evaluation, I met Luz and we traveled to the jornada. The group from Toronto had converted offices in the headquarters of a local nongovernmental organization (NGO) into exam rooms, and we received a number and waited in line. While we waited, Luz decided to pass the time fruitfully by furthering our ongoing relationship of exchange. Gina Ulysse (2002) poignantly reminds us that during fieldwork, ethnographers are not the only ones with projects and that race, class, and gender differences can translate into attempts to remake the anthropologists into more respectable women. My status as a thirty-one-year-old, unmarried, and childless woman was of obvious concern to women I interviewed, who were mothers, the vast majority of whom were married. The women pitied me not only because I was living alone, which they assumed must have made me feel bad, but because of my single social status. I found this exhausting. Luz, as a married woman with children, had successfully solved what she perceived was a major problem I faced. In appreciation of my effort to accompany her to the jornada, Luz consoled me on my unmarried and childless state. She pointed out that I should not despair because I was so full of potential—I was attractive, I was kind. She told me that life worked in mysterious ways and that there was still time for me to find someone to share it with and be fulfilled. While I did listen to Luz, I tried to put her at ease by marshaling a defense. I told her that in my country, people marry later. I had not even finished my degree. I did want to have children and was still optimistic that it would happen someday. She seemed glad that I was not depressed, but she also viewed my biological clock as ticking much faster than I seemed to.

Finally, we were called into an office with an examination table. We greeted the doctor, who sat behind her desk and started a background interview. Luz talked while I translated. Eventually the doctor asked Luz to get up on the exam table so she could do a physical exam. Luz removed her underwear, loosed the belt around her skirt, and lay down on the table. The doctor moved to the end of the table between Luz's legs, and I stood at her head, still translating. The briefest of exams revealed immediately that Luz's uterus was indeed problematically hanging out of her vagina. After the exam, we sat down in front of the desk again, where the doctor pulled out a plastic model of a uterus and vagina to explain the surgery she thought Luz needed. What I understood, and thus relayed to Luz, was that the surgeon would cut the uterus above Luz's cervix and then tack up the remaining flesh so that it stayed inside. Luz thought about it for a moment and declared that, given the amount

xii

of suffering her prolapsed uterus had caused her, she wanted to undergo the surgery.

We then left the surgeon and went to another station, where we were given instructions on when and where to show up, as well as on what we had to bring the day of the surgery. The jornada had rented a private Catholic hospital in the nearby provincial capital. Luz would have her surgery on the first day that they began to operate on people. She would need to arrive early in the morning and was expected to be finished with her surgery around lunch. She would need to stay two to three or maybe even four days, depending on how her surgery went and how she felt. During that time, we had to bring her necessities, like food and toiletries.

On the morning of the surgery, I accompanied Luz, her husband, and their older children to the city. We walked to the hospital that the jornada had rented and found a bustle of people at work. Luz was processed in triage and given a hospital bracelet and gown. Her family carefully packed her *huipil* and *corte* into a bag to keep them safe.[4] She was assigned a bed that had been placed in the hallway due to the overcrowding that the jornada caused. We waited for her to be taken to the operating room, and around lunchtime, once her surgery was completed and she was awake, she was wheeled back into the hall. Her family was able to keep her company and care for her while she convalesced. She stayed the full four days before she was discharged. Luz's surgery and her stay at the jornada ostensibly went well.

At this point, we were all pleased with the outcome of these events, each for our own reason. Obviously, Luz was thrilled not to have to deal with her prolapsed uterus anymore. Her family was glad that her suffering had been alleviated and that she was able to get the medical attention she needed for the cost of transport, food, and care, all of which were within their ability to provide. I was pleased that I was able to connect her to a resource that she wanted as well as to help her navigate it.

Knowing that the obstetrician was a practicing surgeon whom I could have seen in other circumstances for my own care reassured me. I undoubtedly found the experience of attending the mission more familiar in many ways than that of witnessing the daily care that I saw administered in public hospitals and clinics in Guatemala. For example, it was rare at that time to encounter an obstetrician at public hospitals, unless in the capital city, and it was even rarer for an obstetrician to be a woman, as this mission volunteer was. The surgeon had also used a plastic anatomy model of the female reproductive system to explain the procedure. I had not seen this sort of explanation accompanied by didactic materials in any of the clinics and hospitals that I had visited or observed during my research. I appreciated the plastic model and thought that it, along with the obstetrician's explanation, helped me understand the particularities of the surgery. All in all, this familiarity inspired my trust.

In hindsight, my familiarity with this experience undoubtedly indicated its unfamiliarity to Luz. Because doctors in Guatemala's public hospitals were overburdened with patients, they did not have time to explain the physiology of a condition, and patients did not ask for this kind of explanation. Biology was not a standard part of the school curriculum in Guatemala, and most Indigenous people where I lived did not complete high school at this time, perhaps rendering the plastic anatomy models that were so familiar to me inscrutable. But I do not know. Luz never mentioned the plastic model.

Two weeks after Luz's surgery, a child came to my house and asked me to visit Luz. When I arrived at her house, I found her in bed and in pain. Her family told me that when she first returned, Luz was fine, and then she started not to feel well. Now, she felt weak and could no longer walk. We were all immediately worried about the surgery.

The next day, I had to return to the provincial capital to go to the public hospital, and while there, I stopped by the emergency room to talk to the doctor on duty about Luz's case. I wanted him to say, "Oh, this is probably just an insignificant infection. Take this antibiotic," or "Bring her in, and we'll take a look." Instead, I found the conversation quite pointed. "What sort of surgery did she have?" he asked. I explained that she had been suffering from prolapse and that the surgeon had removed her uterus and tacked up what remained. "What method? What tests did they do before the surgery? Were there any complications during the surgery? What records do you have?" I was taken aback by the litany of questions. Prior to this discussion, I thought that I had a pretty good idea of Luz's medical procedure and her current symptoms. But I had no answer for the types of questions being asked. Luz did not leave the jornada with a case file or any other information to help us determine what had happened to her. I tried to push back and ask if it was just an infection that could be easily treated. The doctor seemed disappointed in me. He said that it could be an infection but that it could also be something else. To illustrate his point, he told me what had happened to another Indigenous woman, just like to Luz, whose family decided to seek surgical care from a jornada. Like Luz, she qualified in the screening and returned from her surgery believing that her problem had been resolved. While the surgery did address her immediate issue, it created another, worse, problem—aggressively growing cervical cancer. During the surgery, the team had cut through that woman's cervix, which, unbeknownst to the mission surgeons, was cancerous. While the cervical cancer had previously been slow-growing and asymptomatic, after the surgery, it grew more aggressively. The woman ended up dying from cancer shortly after the diagnosis.

After that anecdote came a lecture: patients, he told me, turn to jornadas for quick and cheap treatment of their conditions. The problem is that some conditions are complex, and quick and cheap treatment of complex conditions can be not only ineffective but dangerous. Doctors at the hospital know that patients in the public hospital have minimal access to health care. They therefore require patients to undergo extensive presurgical tests, including blood work, X-rays, and in the case of gynecological surgeries, Pap smears. Because improving cervical cancer outcomes has been at the forefront of the Guatemala Ministry of Health's reproductive health goals since the turn of the millennium, no gynecological surgeries happen without a Pap smear. When Luz had her surgery, very few women in Sololá would ever have had a Pap smear. Within the public system, all Pap smears had to be sent to Guatemala City for analysis, and there was an inevitable delay in processing the sample. Pap smears, the doctor explained, were part of normal medical protocols in North America, where a surgeon would hesitate to treat a patient who had never had one. Why, then, he asked me, would that same surgeon come to Guatemala and be willing to operate on a patient who had never had one? He then told me to find out what had happened to Luz.

I spent the few days after that encounter in detective mode trying to recover whatever information I could about Luz's surgery. Through the expatriate community in the town where I found the original flier, I was easily able to track down some contact information for the organization that had hosted the jornada. Organization staffers told me that patient records were kept in English and thus stored abroad with the medical team; they also gave me the contact information of the jornada organizer in Toronto, with whom I began a series of email and telephone exchanges. I sent her Luz's full name and the date of her surgery. Within a week, she replied, but not with the information that I sought. The records had been brought back to Toronto and immediately stored in her basement. However, she was unable to give me any information about Luz's surgery because, in the subsequent week, her basement had been flooded and the records destroyed.

While I was trying to get information about what had happened to Luz, Luz's family decided to hire a retired nurse who lived in their village. The nurse prescribed antibiotics and came to Luz's house every afternoon to give her intravenous fluids. Within a week, Luz's condition improved. After two, she was up and walking. When her suffering ebbed, my relief was palpable.

I considered Luz's case closed until many years later, when I received a desperate phone call from my friend Barbara, a North American who lived in same village as Luz. Luz had asked her to call me because her prolapse had returned. "What happened at that jornada?" Barbara asked me. Luz told Barbara that the surgeons had cut out her uterus. "Then what's hanging down between her legs now?" Barbara demanded. Luz was suffering and confused. Barbara was upset. I was home in Canada. The records were still nowhere to be found.

Unfortunately, the story ends here. Luz is still alive, but it is hard to know exactly what happened in the jornada. Different doctors have told me different theories. Rather than speculate, I think that the ambiguous denouement of this saga represents realistically how Luz, Barbara, and I have come to feel about it.

This story became the origin story for this book not because it was my first encounter with missions, or even because it was enduring, but because these events brought medical missions into the center of my personal and scholarly attention. At that time, my research was on global maternal health agendas; I was already working with women, like Luz, in villages, and I was also deeply engaged in the public health system— exploring population health interventions to decrease maternal mortality and to transform clinical care. But my experience with Luz led me to engage my medical colleagues in the Guatemalan public health system—with whom I normally only talked about obstetric care—about this case.

I was surprised by the vehemence with which my medical colleagues expressed their dislike for medical missions.[5] A major part of their disdain stemmed from their experiences dealing with mission cases that had gone wrong, and indeed I heard a litany of horror stories with poor endings for patients. They repeatedly told me that North American doctors do not know how to practice medicine here.

At the time, I found the rejection of jornadas on this basis confusing. I had spent a lot of the time with my Guatemalan colleagues in trainings and reviews geared toward importing emergency obstetric-care protocols developed by "experts" at the World Health Organization (WHO) in Geneva into the Guatemalan health system. Ironically, many of the foreign-mission doctors arriving to Guatemala could have easily been among the cadre of professionals writing WHO manuals; many were senior physicians from top metropolitan learning hospitals holding privileged positions with the kinds of grants and social capital that produced "expert" medical knowledge. If foreign doctors from the North did not know how to practice medicine in Guatemala, why were my colleagues in the public system in Guatemala so amenable to importing "best practices" and consulting WHO manuals to provide better emergency obstetric care? What was the difference between foreign-led global maternal-health initiatives and foreign-led medical missions? What made my colleagues covet one and excoriate the other? What made one seem so useful and beneficial and the other irresponsible at best and dangerous at worst? These questions started me on the road to seriously considering medical missions as a topic of scholarly inquiry.

Eight years after bringing Luz to get surgery, I submitted a grant proposal to take a deeper look at medical missions in Sololá, which appeared to me to have grown in number and influence in the intervening years. That research not only took me back to the public hospital in Sololá to talk to my health professional colleagues in Guatemala but also put me in conversation with a new group of colleagues—those traveling from the North and staffing the missions. After several years of data collection, I sat down to write this book.

My first step in writing this book was to go back through years of field notes in an attempt to piece together what had happened to Luz. After writing a draft of her story, I tried to pick apart the narrative to map it onto the themes of what I thought I had learned about missions. However, the more I wrote, the more I suspected that something was missing in my approach. My material felt distant and bounded, while my experiences had been profound and omnipresent.

For me, this disjuncture between my early drafts and my experiences was captured perfectly by Luz's case. The exercise of thematic mapping led me to write the specifics of Luz's story, then analyze abstractly the details of her case to show how they illustrated important generalities about medical missions. This process led me to focus on contextualizing medical missions within the landscape of global health interventions that occur in places like Sololá.[6] This approach also caused me to question whether missions are helpful vis-à-vis important contemporary issues of universal access to care and the strengthening of health care systems. Yet when I happen to wake up in the middle of the night and my thoughts start running, Luz's case often pops into my mind. In those moments, I am never drawn to consider what I can generalize from Luz's story; rather, I am always mulling over my decisions. Did I do the right thing? Would it have been better for Luz if I had just taken the interview, given her the soap, and left?

I brought Luz to that jornada not because I puzzled over the consequences of doing or not doing so but because when I saw that announcement taped to the telephone pole, telling her about the jornada immediately felt like the right thing for me to do. I asked something of her (to grant the interview), and then she asked something of me (to keep my eyes open for opportunities). When I saw the jornada announcement, it immediately seemed like a good opportunity. Bringing Luz an opportunity only solidified our exchange relationship and encouraged her to consider how she could continue to help me. While we waited on the bench at the NGO to see the mission doctor, Luz tried to counsel me. She had successfully navigated her transition from girl to woman, making a good match, leaving her household, and eventually surrounding herself with loving children and a devoted husband. From her perspective, I had not fared as well; at thirty-one, I was still unmarried and childless. She saw a need. She found a fix. She tried to use her experience to help me navigate unfamiliar waters. I did the same. I felt confident bringing her to doctors who were licensed and practicing in Toronto—the same sorts of surgeons that I would see if I had her problem. I imagined that they would operate successfully to repair Luz's prolapse. And that is what happened. Until it was not. While the consequences of Luz's "help" were certainly less disastrous than mine, in many senses our motivations were the same. We both wanted to live the types of lives in which we were people who acted to help others. Luz's story became the origin story of this book because it made me reconsider how this desire to live an ethical life forms a cornerstone of global health practices.

# Introduction

*Intimate Connections and the Making of Global Health*

This book is motivated by a central question: What can we learn about global health when our intimate connections to our own actions become the locus of inquiry? Considering short-term medical missions (STMM) as a model of global health practice, the book focuses on experiences of mission volunteers, including myself. Luz's story from the prologue, of receiving care from volunteer doctors on a medical mission from Canada but then experiencing complications once the volunteers were long gone, with no records left behind of what they had done, illustrates how I arrived at this question. When I started writing this book, I attempted to understand what happened to Luz in terms of wider structures of inequality. Nevertheless, even as I wrote about those wider structures, I was preoccupied by other questions: What kind of person would I be if I had pretended that my obligation to Luz ended with that bar of soap? If I had just given her the soap, nodded at her request to keep an eye out for opportunities, and forgotten all about her? Later, as I began to make sense of my own experiences volunteering at STMMs, my focus was again drawn to the personal and intimate. My own moments of taking action, like bringing Luz to the jornada or helping to treat particular patients, were what I found most compelling. My intent in acting mattered to me. How I felt about my actions in hindsight mattered to me. Whether my actions had contributed to helping or harming really mattered to me. While connections between feelings and actions had been a focus of scholarly work on humanitarian action and development work, this interest had not filtered into critical scholarship on global health. I decided to switch tacks and see what would happen if I made those intimate connections my focus. To wit, the intimate connections I explore in this book are not about relationships with others. Rather, they are about our innermost relationships with ourselves as we each reflect on the kind of person we want to be and what actions we will take in order to lead us to the type of life that we think of as good.

Despite a lack of attention, the "global health domain," a phrase I use to refer to multiplicities of actions and practices that people undertake in the name of "global health," lends itself to thinking about people's connections to their own actions.[1] Practices in this domain frequently involve people going outside their own home geographies to act with the intent of improving health and promoting health equity. Because global health work aims to improve the world, it becomes part of many people's ethical lives.[2] Furthermore, many people see global health work as ethically important work and, by extension, working in global health as doing something good with their lives. The domain of global health is, therefore, steeped with people wanting to do the right thing.[3]

Anthropologists have heartily engaged this impulse in global health by pointing out that many attempts to do the right thing ultimately worsen the very conditions they were meant to address in the first place. To be sure, ethnographies from myriad locales have demonstrated how agendas ignoring structural inequalities that create the "need" for global health interventions at best do nothing and at worst exacerbate the difficult conditions of many systemically oppressed groups (Benton, 2015b; Fan, 2021; Kalofonos, 2021; Suh, 2021). This is all the truer for humanitarian health responses motivated by a crisis (Allen, 2015; Jézéquel, 2015; Wagner, 2015). While connecting inequitable structures to people's poor health is a major contribution of contemporary anthropology, this approach tends to sideline both considerations of an individual's intent to do good and feelings about what they did. What has mattered instead is the on-the-ground impact of what was done.

This book does something different. It asks, What we can learn if we take seriously the good intentions undergirding global health action? How does a person come to feel that their action was the right (or wrong) thing to do? Indeed, I argue that taking seriously the intent to do good is instrumental to understanding why contemporary global health looks the way it does today. Focusing on the influence of our own reflections on actions we take to live the type of life that we think of as good can nudge us to think differently about global health action and global health programming.

As I began to focus on interior, intimate experiences, I came to realize that *visceral ethics* frequently underwrites global health practice and thus helps explain it. I define visceral ethics as the idea that one uses gut feelings to validate the ethical nature of our own action; that is, if something feels viscerally "good," that feeling allows one to judge that their action is, in fact, good. In subsequent chapters, I show how and why visceral ethics can be an integral part of global health practitioners' experiences, including mitigating the decontextualization inherent to global work, and therefore an integral part of how practitioners come to understand those experiences. Ultimately, I contend that acknowledging visceral ethics is important to understanding action in the global health domain. This driving force of meaning-making for practitioners fundamentally propels global health activities and encounters, like short-term medical missions, in the contemporary world. By driving actions, visceral ethics can also drive the problematic consequences of global health engagement, reinforcing existing inequities and producing "unintended" harmful consequences (Berry, 2010; Closser, 2010; Kamat, 2013; Powis, 2022).

Visceral ethics pertains to what anthropologists have called "ordinary ethics" (Das, 2010, 2012, 2015; Lambek, 2010). Ordinary ethics attends to ethics as emergent and immediate rather than contingent on articulated norms and rules that typically form the basis of philosophical ethics. The anthropologist Veena Das's (2012:139) analysis of everyday life demonstrates "the natural expression of ethics," as people navigate complicated social situations, without, for example, alienating or offending their interlocutors. Das looks to such complex navigations to highlight the ordinariness of ethics—indeed ethical practice is part of being human and social (Das, 2015). She also emphasizes that this sort of anthropological inquiry is not about stated rules and norms but rather about the "habits and customs that form the texture of everyday life" (2012:139). Following Das, my analysis of visceral ethics derives from examinations of the everyday lives of global health practitioners and their attempts to do the right thing as they navigate global health practice.

As alluded to in the definition, visceral ethics also attends to an immediacy of feelings that practicing in the global health domain can engender. In considering the role of affect in giving rise to the world in which we live, the social anthropologist Naisargi Dave (2012) argues that the potential of affect derives from its "embryonic"-ness, painting affect as nascent or immature. Dave emphasizes that affect is persuasive in its "intensity" yet exists outside of articulated, fixed, or "assimilated" aspects of the world. As such, affect defines "the formative but embryonic aspects of what moves us in the world" (Dave, 2012:9). Dave's (2011, 2012) point that affect is something not yet fully formed is central to its importance. As she demonstrates, affect can be instrumental in spaces and moments that are wholly constructed in the minds or imaginations of individuals. Drawing on one of Dave's examples, a person in New Delhi can crave to live in a world as both an Indian and a lesbian, whose love for her partner is socially accepted (or even embraced), despite the fact that this is currently impossible. In this way, Dave demonstrates how affect can function in spaces incommensurable with the "real" world. Through visceral ethics, I link the creative power of affect firmly to practitioners' meaning-making regarding good moral action.[4] Dave's work shows us how affect can make practitioners' experiences of the intensity characteristic of global health work powerfully important and formative. Yet it also shows how visceral ethics does not need to be commensurable with outcomes produced in the "real" world. Rather, visceral ethics allows practitioners to use their own judgments, based on their own limited understandings of the contexts in which they work, to determine what is right or good.

## Anthropology of Global Health: A Structural Analysis of Justice?

Anthropological scholarship has made a sizeable and unique contribution to the study of global health through ethnography (Ji & Cheng, 2021; MacDonald, 2017). As the medical anthropologist Stacy Pigg (2013) has pointed out, while global health is typically a field that is characterized by "doing" and doing it now, ethnography as a mode of research enfranchises extensive time for engagement and reflection (what Pigg refers to as "sitting"). Anthropologists join other disciplines taking the field of global health itself as our object of study, separating ourselves from predominant approaches "invested in developing models . . . of optimal interventions and in identifying and evaluating programs that supposedly 'work'" (Biehl, 2016:129). The medical anthropologists Craig Janes and Kitty Corbett (2009:169), however, claim that even in cases in which anthropologists study others "doing" something, the goal is "to reduce global health inequities and contribute to the development of sustainable and salutogenic sociocultural, political, and economic systems" (cf. Pigg, 2013). Janes and Corbett's remarks point to a moral underpinning commonly found in the anthropology of global health. The medical anthropologists João Biehl and Adriana Petryna (2013) provide insight into what this moral underpinning might look like: anthropology is distinguished in its contribution to global health by the practice of putting "people . . . first." Indeed, our disciplinary emphasis on linguistic fluency, participant observation, extensive field seasons, and long-term engagement with place means that anthropologists have front-row seats to observe the everyday lives of people. So while much of the field is taken up by the voices of experts, planners, and other high-level folks doing global health work, ethnographies tend to provide one of the few venues that highlight the perspectives of recipients as "targets," or subjects of global health efforts.

My own work has been heavily shaped by these thematic divides. It has tended to cohere around a dominant theoretical orientation concerning dynamics of power relations between the macro, meso, and micro levels. Biehl (2016) offers a more sophisticated rendering of this orientation. He envisions the contribution of ethnography to global health as "charting the lives of individuals and institutions over time, chronicling people's varied interpretations of their conditions, all the while denaturalizing operational categories and illuminating the concrete ways meso- and macro-level actors impinge on local worlds and become part of global orders" (2016:135). Work in the anthropology of global health, perhaps because of its moral underpinnings, tends to emphasize how institutions, bureaucracies, categories, and so on shape action and experience. Per Biehl, such a focus has allowed us to illuminate not only inequities themselves but also the novel and naturalized modes through which inequities are propagated.

My own scholarship on global health has been tightly bound to these moral underpinnings. I am suspicious of approaches to global health work and interventions purporting to remediate health inequities without working on (or referring to) the structures that give rise to these inequities. Further, I am skeptical of interventions that draw on longstanding power relations without reflecting on how these power relations not only benefit "experts" but also maintain the inequities that drew aid in the first place. I am supportive of interventions seeking to eliminate the causes of inequities and skeptical of more immediate approaches that address only the outcomes of these causes. These concerns were central to my analysis when I began this project. As a result, initially when I began writing this book, I tried to interpret Luz's story on the basis of the structural inequalities that gave rise to her experience. Doing so reflected my training and its moral underpinnings.

Scholars of anthropology and ethics have wrangled with the relative importance of individuals and their experiences to the worlds in which they live. Following the sociologist Zygmunt Bauman (1988), the anthropologist James Laidlaw (2013) referred to what he considers an overemphasis on structure as the anthropology "of unfreedom," signaling anthropologists' lack of theoretical interest in individual agency. Similarly, in an inquiry into the uptake of virtue ethics in anthropology, Cheryl Mattingly (2012) focuses on the overwhelming allegiance in anthropology to "third-person" accounts, which are accounts that emphasize the role of higher-level phenomena in structuring individual action. She cites the later writing of the French sociologist Michel Foucault as influencing anthropological scholarship to view individual, everyday practices as enactments of larger discourses. Mattingly takes the anthropologist Saba Mahmood's (2005) study of the women's piety movement in Egypt as an exemplar. Mahmood attends to the everyday mechanisms through which her participants cultivate piety; yet Mahmood follows Foucault in her position that what is of interest is relating subject-making to larger discourses that enfranchise particular subject positions.

Are these critiques useful for an anthropology of global health? We live in an increasingly inequitable world. Exposing the articulations of power that underwrite inequity is a necessary component to pursuing justice. However, our attention to structure might be foreclosing a close analysis of action or agency. Backing away from exposing structures of power as our object of inquiry might seem frighteningly naïve and, frankly, useless for an anthropology of global health. However, just because anthropologists of global health have become proficient at one very necessary mode of scholarship does not obviate the value of other modes.

This has been both a major lesson for me in writing this book and what I see as one of the main contributions of my exploration of visceral ethics. I began this project the same way I began my other scholarship on global health: with an analysis propelled by notions of justice. I was, therefore, focused on how short-term medical missions leave structures of power unaddressed, as well as how they arguably reenact those structures. Due to what I perceived as lack of serious attention to dismantling inequities, I considered short-term medical missions unrelated to the pursuit of justice and, because of this, never considered a theoretical framework that might analyze mission work as a form of ethical action. Subsequently, however, I realized that my own experience upholds Pigg's (2013:128) argument that insisting on theoretical frames privileging the pursuit of justice "foreclose[s] directions of inquiry that might emerge through ethnographic discovery by prematurely containing what should be investigated."[5] As Pigg suggests, this pursuit of justice "foreclose[d]" my inquiry. Though I left missions where I volunteered feeling like the work I had done was integrally connected to important ethical action, I ignored this feeling when embarking on my writing. Furthermore, I considered my own preoccupation with how my actions actually played out in the world (e.g., Was Luz *actually* better off?) as personal and not illustrative of the dynamics of global health. When I finally began to experiment with the idea of centering my own and others' intimate experiences, I quickly realized that I could not both do this and privilege ideas of justice that were prominent in my past work. A focus on justice in global health is intertwined with a disciplinary preference to view the intimate as subordinate to the structural. This made it impossible to hold justice and intimacy in balance.[6] Because an exploration of the intimate was fertile, new ground, I decided to prioritize it. I therefore took Kathleen Stewart's (2007:4) advice to let go of "bottom-line arguments about 'bigger' structures and underlying causes " and instead focus on "the complex and uncertain [things] that fascinate because they . . . exert a pull on us." Theoretically, this book shifts away from structural analyses of justice and is instead premised on the idea that taking seriously people's intimate experiences and thoughts about their own actions can tell us something new and important about global health. The people with whom I am specifically concerned are those who come together to organize and staff short-term medical missions.

## DIY Global Health and the Ethical Lives of Volunteers

Short-term medical missions are part of the ever-growing and important sector of contemporary global health that I call "do-it-yourself (DIY) global health."[7] To date, scholarship on global health has attended to more formal engagements, typically involving structures created nationally and internationally by organizations that have a footprint. DIY global health functions outside of formal host-country systems (e.g., ministries of health). Actions undertaken through DIY global health have little accountability, and when these endeavors have concluded, they leave virtually no documentation of having been present. Though DIY global health is ephemeral, tens of thousands of people become involved in some form of DIY global health, such as medical missions, every year (Lasker, 2016).

Short-term medical missions, one example of DIY global health, have escaped easy definition due to variations in practice (Sykes, 2014). Nevertheless, the jornadas I studied frequently had certain commonalities.[8] All of the missions I studied were associated with NGOs. Often they would need to co-opt an existing space and adapt it to fit their activities. For example, Luz and I went to the headquarters of a local NGO for her initial examination; the doctor who evaluated her had set up an examining table in one of the offices. When it was time for her surgery, the jornada had rented a small, private hospital, including operating-room time and gurneys for recovery. The missions I studied were staffed by licensed, North American medical practitioners, including different types of surgeons, anesthesiologists, eye doctors, family doctors, midwives, and medical imaging specialists. Missions were short-term programs, unfolding over the course of a few weeks or less. In addition, no medical practitioner received money for participating in the jornadas that I studied; rather, jornada volunteers had to pay for their trips, usually worked during unpaid leave or vacation time, and covered a share of the medical supplies needed to give care.[9] Jornadas were funded through some combination of fundraising and paying out of pocket. Additionally, the constraints on staffing jornadas meant that many clinicians took on work that an assistant might have done at home, such as taking vitals, cleaning equipment, or going out to the waiting room to call the next patient.

Scholarship focused on humanitarian workers, particularly Western volunteers, provides the most insight into people who engage in DIY global health work, like medical missions.[10] The sociologist Judith Lasker (2016) conducted 119 interviews with international medical volunteers from the US who characterized their motivations for engaging this work along a range of altruism (e.g., helping others in need) to self-interest (e.g., giving a retired medical practitioner a purpose). Anthropological approaches to humanitarianism have discarded the assumption that humanitarian work is transparently explained by the suffering of others and the volunteers' alleviation of such suffering (Fassin, 2011). Indeed, the anthropologist Lissa Malkki (2015) urges us to consider what needs humanitarian action might fulfill in aid workers themselves. For example, Finnish knitters who make gifts for children abroad find meaning in feeling connected to a world beyond their own.[11] Moreover, Malkki show that professionals are drawn to international placements that help them "lose themselves in the intensity of sustained demanding work" (Malkki, 2015:11). Malkki's insight that exploration of the self is essential to a complete rendering of volunteering has been instrumental in guiding me toward an exploration of visceral ethics.

Furthermore, ethnographies of Western volunteers have highlighted how volunteering is, as the anthropologist Britt Halvorson (2020:152) phrases it, "an activity saturated with emotion"; the high emotion stemming from the love and care volunteers put into their work is endemic to volunteering. The anthropologist Erica Bornstein (2012) describes an almost addictive fervor expressed by Westerners volunteering in India; volunteering generated feelings so persuasive and fulfilling that volunteers gave up their past professions and tried to convince others to join them. Where might such fervor come from? The anthropologists Andrea Muehlebach (2012) and Vincanne Adams (2013b) each propose a political-economic analysis of a neoliberal state focused on privatization and profit, where volunteers take up the slack of a withdrawing or absent state.[12] Acceptance of this downloading of care is made palatable through a veneration of compassion (Muehlebach, 2012). My approach to this question, however, is more in line with Halvorson's (2020). Halvorson ties affect to ethical lives of volunteers. Rather than focusing on discourse or structures that produce affect, she encourages us to consider the role of affect in producing "interactive moments through which [volunteers'] ethical lives are defined and negotiated" (Halvorson, 2020:160).

The anthropologist Webb Keane's (2016:20) clarification of "ethical lives" as concerned with "how one should live and what kind of person one should be" is instructive for thinking about what draws volunteers to STMMs. A fundamental contention of this book is that volunteers are drawn to DIY global health opportunities because they align with the type of life a volunteer believes they should live. As the anthropologist Betsey Brada (2023:2) argues, in the contemporary world, global health is widely perceived "to generate goodness in those who participate in it." Working at a medical mission is therefore taking action consonant with the type of person that the volunteer wants to be. Volunteering for a medical mission is ethical action or action that is "oriented with reference to values and ends that are not in turn defined as the means to some further ends" (Keane, 2016:4) and thus central to a volunteer's ethical life.

My approach to ethical action is centered on what the anthropologist Anand Pandian and the historian Daud Ali (2010) term "pre-humanistic" ethics—that is, traditions that highlight the important role of what I call an individual's intimate connection with their own action rather than a focus on externally articulated norms and rules to judge action. I draw heavily on virtue ethics, centered on what the anthropologist Edward F. Fischer (2014:2) describes as the Aristotelian quest to live "the good life" and related to "the power to construct a life that one values." Virtue ethics is premised on the idea that I cultivate my own virtues by practicing what I value (generosity, humility, honesty, etc.).[13] In my case, taking Luz to the jornada reflected my values of responsibility (I initiated our exchange relationship) and trustworthiness (I wanted to follow through on what I said I would do). In general, then, I consider the actions volunteers undertake in the global health domain as their attempts to live good lives. For the medical missioners I worked with, volunteering for a jornada is an ethical action; jornadas are spaces where clinicians can practice doing the types of good they value. Within this project, then, attention to external judgments (like yours or mine) about whether actions are right or wrong are secondary. Instead, my inquiry focuses on volunteers' intent to do good and how this intent translates into feelings about whether the actions they took did good.

My focus on North Americans as organizers and workers at short-term medical missions certainly influences the concepts of ethical action and the intimate dispositions explored in this book. Pandian and Ali (2010) remind us that contemporary ideas of ethical practice (e.g., going to Guatemala to do surgeries for two weeks), as well as embodied responses to working in global health domains, emerge from our historical pasts. For example, Pandian (2009) shows us that the way in which Kallar people of southern India strive to cultivate both themselves and their land remains firmly tied to ideas of development and progress shaped by a colonial past. Indeed Pandian (2009:5) indicates how the low status of the Kallar caste and colonial projects to reform Kallar people and their "crooked" ways underwrite contemporary perceptions of "the nature of Kallar selfhood . . . as a moral and ethical problem." The "enduring weight of colonial subjugation" is also evident in the fact that the Kallar can and do fail in morally righteous cultivation both of the land and of themselves. We see the same stakes of failure evident in Das's (2012) examples of everyday ethical lives. Das's interlocutors have, in a sense, trained their whole lives to face daily ethical dilemmas. Their actions, and explanations of those actions, betray an encyclopedic understanding of the myriad factors contributing to their decision-making. Not only are the actors and situations tied tightly to time and place, but a constant threat of loss or failure accompanies a wrong move (Mattingly, 2014).

Pandian's and Das's examples draw to the fore how ethical lives must be anchored not only in particular times and places but also to social locations. The relative privilege of North Americans who organize and serve in jornadas has left a clear watermark on this book.[14] Just as judgment and the threat of failure are an integral part of the lives of Pandian and Ali's (2010) participants, the ability of North Americans to work unjeopardized (and frequently unlicensed) in geographic areas where they have minimal contextual knowledge speaks to privilege inherent in their social locations.[15] This privilege also enables notions of visceral ethics. In the absence of deep contextual understandings, STMM volunteers rely heavily on visceral ethics to underwrite their actions as virtuous, and they are able to do so because their social location accords them latitude to judge and define their own actions in ways that are unavailable to them in their professional work at home.

Proposing visceral ethics as a theoretical force in global health shifts my analysis from an examination of structures of inequality. It follows anthropological scholarship on ethics that has sought to rebalance the relative importance of structure in producing action. For many scholars, this rebalancing means attending (for some, almost exclusively) to the experiences and reflexivity of individuals in particular moments. Yet Keane (2014b:451) cautions that such an overemphasis on "internal states" is ultimately as artificially polarizing as our current (overly) structural approach and that we must "situate . . . ethical life within a social world without going back to . . . social determinism." While I agree with Keane, the details of what constitutes a sufficient middle ground are unsettled, and thus I want to address up front how this goal of rebalancing has influenced my ethnography. Given the sparse attention to experiences, feelings, and particularities of individual persons in building both theory and our understandings of global health, at this juncture I find it important to privilege reflexivity and intimate experiences over structures.[16] In the following section, I describe what this has meant methodologically for my project.

## Research Design

To obtain funding for this project, I framed my research into medical missions as an inquiry into DIY global health. Jornadas were fairly unique among the myriad foreign organizations in Sololá that worked on women's health, as they rebuffed the dominant development orthodoxy of partnership with host-country organizations (e.g., the ministry of health). They were intentionally small and barebones, preferring to frontload their resources into service delivery and rely on volunteer labor for sustainability. My proposed project explored the ways in which jornada volunteers conceptualized modernity and how these conceptualizations shaped their engagement in development. To capitalize on my areas of interest, I focused on jornadas that came to Sololá and worked in the domain of reproductive health. To gain a more holistic understanding of jornadas, I decided not only to do fieldwork within short-term medical missions myself but to focus simultaneously on how jornadas were contextualized and understood within Guatemala. I wanted to know how professional Guatemalans thought about STMMs in their country, how STMMs linked up with NGOs, and how the publics served by missions viewed them.

During fieldwork, what I did and how I did it were tailored to these original objectives. Nonetheless, as I outlined earlier, I realized that this framing obscured my own intimate experiences. When I decided that my book should focus on precisely what had been obscured, I ended up having to become creative in how to (re)analyze my data. This section therefore details the data-collection methods that I used, geared toward my original purpose, and speaks to the transitions I made in reanalyzing my data toward issues of visceral ethics that emerged, inductively, after fieldwork.

As alluded to in the prologue, despite the fact that STMMs were not the focus of my research in Sololá until 2012, the ethnographic corpus that underwrites this book stems from my long-term relationship with Sololá, Guatemala, where I have worked since 1999. My first interaction with a medical mission occurred in 2000, and I have field notes touching on the topic since then. During the winter of 2013, my family and I moved back to Sololá for a five-month field season; I also made two shorter return trips by myself. I used my initial time in Sololá to interview Guatemalan health care professionals, all of whom worked in conjunction with the Guatemalan ministry responsible for health.[17] I started interviewing professionals in particular capacities who I thought would be important to my study and then asked those individuals to recommend others who might have important perspectives on my topic. I explored their opinions of STMMs, how missions related to or impeded ministry goals, why several areas of government were cracking down on mission activity, and the difference between foreign medical activities promulgated by the WHO and STMMs. Ultimately, I spoke in-depth to eleven Guatemalan health professionals, some of whom were engaged in providing clinical care in hospitals or the health districts and others who worked in administration or as consultants. This interview process also led me to speak to a representative from the Guatemalan College of Physicians and Surgeons, as well as to a former high-ranking ministry official, both of whom I met in Guatemala City.

Much of my research activity was also dictated by my continued interest in reproductive health. Medical missions operate in many different domains of medicine; I attempted to streamline my approach by concentrating on surgical interventions in reproductive health. This focus led me back to the public hospital in Sololá (where I had spent time a decade before doing research on the Safe Motherhood Initiative) to consider why certain women sought care there, while others turned to jornadas. I interviewed eight women who were seeking treatment in the hospital, waiting in outpatient care to visit gynecologists or recuperating in postoperation recovery wards. I also spent time tracking down and studying the handwritten surgery registry books at the public hospital dating from 2008 to 2012. These books are the only places that accurately detail the surgeries performed in the operating theaters of the public hospital. I hoped that getting a better understanding of surgical capacity and production in Sololá would help answer questions about whether jornadas addressed an outstanding surgical need. After entering this data in Excel, I realized that there was no discernable pattern regarding the number or type of surgeries related to women's reproductive health that were performed. This complicated my attempts to pin down the feasible number of surgeries that could be done. I showed graphs of the Excel data to health-professional interviewees to begin a second conversation about constraints on hospital capacity and ways to define surgical need in populations.

My focus on reproductive health also shaped my approach to short-term medical missions. First, when selecting potential clinician interviewees, I searched the internet for medical professionals who disclosed volunteer stints in Sololá performing gynecological surgeries. I also tried to track down individuals who were involved with a particular NGO that had begun working in the hospital in Sololá and had also done gynecological surgeries. After accompanying jornadas, I interviewed clinicians whom I had met while working with them at a jornada. Ultimately, I interviewed nineteen volunteer clinicians. Sixteen of these interviews occurred over Skype; three I conducted in person. I also interviewed twenty-eight patients from medical missions (the vast majority of whom were treated for gynecological surgeries) while they were waiting in recovery to be released.

My interest in medical missions also led me to interview foreigners living long term in Sololá who were involved with jornadas in a variety of ways. Many led NGOs that served as local contacts for North American organizers of medical missions (Berry, 2014). Others served as translators or health care practitioners, creating a variety of entangle-ments in the mission world. Like my focus on health professionals, I began my interviews with a few people who I knew would be important and then asked them to direct me to other important players. Ultimately, I interviewed ten leaders in NGOs and eight foreigners who had other types of relationships with missions. In the chapters that come, I use the generic term "volunteer" to refer to clinicians, NGO organizers, and others involved in jornadas, specifying their roles when necessary.

I consider participant observation and systematic taking of field notes to be cornerstone methodologies in ethnography; they therefore formed an important part of this research. Over the course of this project, I participated as a volunteer in four different medical missions in Sololá. I looked for organizations currently sponsoring jornadas doing gyneco-logical surgeries to volunteer with and asked to serve as a translator for those health professionals who were screening women. In each of these situations, the organizers knew I was conducting research on STMMs and had agreed up front to allow me to volunteer. As soon as I joined the group, I introduced myself and explained my role as a researcher to all other volunteers.

I also participated in my regular life in a town in Sololá, where I have resided periodically for the past twenty years. Coincidentally, during my initial five months, I helped an acquaintance seek out care, and even-tually surgery, for ovarian cysts, a frequent gynecological surgery per-formed at jornadas. Her family ultimately chose to go to an NGO-run hospital rather than a jornada or the public hospital. As the incident unfolded over several weeks, it provided an excellent platform for people in the village where I lived to engage and react to my research. It also provided me with a different perspective from the ones I got from pa-tients at jornadas or the public hospital. Finally, back in Vancouver, I attended a reunion of volunteers who had served together in Guatemala. Field notes not only provided a mode through which I was able to re-cord events but helped me to journal and reflect on what I was learning through my research activities.

Though important, this listing orientation toward data-collection ac-tivities overemphasizes the importance of easily quantifiable indicators, while unintentionally obscuring unquantifiable aspects that were equally important to this ethnography. My long-term relationship with Sololá underwrites and shapes much of the knowledge generated. For example, wrangling with what happened to Luz and how I felt about my own action created a key experience that convinced me that a preoccupation with intimate experience might be just as important to a rendering of contemporary global health as an inquiry into inequitable structures. Furthermore, the quantification of interviewees obscures how conversations were grafted onto existing relationships. I have known for decades many of the people I spoke with in Sololá. Formal interviews were but a waypoint in continual interactions and frequently delved into past conversations and interrogated shared experiences. Likewise, as we will see, working in a medical mission is an intense, shared experience, and the vast majority of the volunteer interviews were with people I served with, conducted after we had returned home. These social connections created an interdependence among my own experiences, my field notes, and my interviews that would not hold if this were a novel project driven by interviewing people I had never met before about *their* experiences.

Although this project was based on many of the same data-collection techniques that I have used in the past, data analysis was quite different for me. The crux of this difference was the importance of what the anthropologist Branwyn Poleykett (2016) refers to as "body knowledge" to my analysis. Poleykett describes how a day job of field research on women glossed as "prostitutes" impacted her experience of getting together with young female friends to go out at night, bringing "pangs of anxiety" every time she fleetingly used her work lens rather than her off-work lens to think about how they would appear. Indeed, Poleykett (2016:483) finds what she calls a "burden of doubled vision [to be] continuous with the experiences of the fieldworkers." She illustrates how the analytical knowledge that she developed—such as the ability to identify a prostitute in a setting and what it means to society if you are a prostitute—became grounded in her body and part of her instinctive reactions. Fieldwork, however, creates possibilities for different sorts of "body-knowledge"—more specifically, it can offer ways to contrast our intellectual knowledge with lived experiences. When those two do not necessarily jibe, fieldwork "exposes that knowing body-subject to certain kinds of uncomfortable existential queries" (Poleykett, 2016:483). Ultimately, then, Poleykett (2016:483) argues that fieldwork "unsettle[s] the particular bodily habitus of the knowing subject."

Poleykett's work has been central to helping me make sense of my own production of knowledge in this research. As discussed earlier, I was confronted with incongruence between what I recovered from intellectual ways of knowing about short-term medical missions and what I uncovered from experiential ones. Neither prepared me for the other. The intellectual registers anchored medical missions as a practice within wider social, historical, political, and intellectual contexts. Yet fieldwork prompted modes of learning that were almost myopically tied to particular moments and my own bodily reactions to those moments. My analytical attention was naturally drawn to the dissonance between what I thought I knew and what I felt. Yet the lack of congruence between knowledge recovered intellectually with that uncovered experientially means that much of my analytical focus was drawn in by trying to synthesize my "double vision." As hard as I tried, I could not make this work.

Ultimately, the analysis of my ethnographic data for this book has been eclectic. I spent a significant amount of time coding the textual corpus of transcripts and field notes that I collected, but my coding took place when I was still focused on recovering theoretical understanding by tracing the role of power in producing inequities. These sorts of understandings appear infrequently in this book, as they were not leading me toward any novel insights. I abandoned the idea of drawing out themes from textual analysis and returned to the drawing board. I drew up a short list of moments in this research that, because of my own intimate experience, as Kathleen Stewart (2007:2) states, "[felt] like *some*thing." I then sought analytical direction among these moments. A conversation with the philosopher whose office is next to mine on campus pushed me toward virtue ethics. It was a short hop from there to anthropology of ethics, where I found eventual inspiration for how to proceed. My chapters are built around significant experiences in my fieldwork, placed in conversation with scholarship that attends to important facets of volunteers' ethical lives.

## All the World's a Stage: Confronting Ideas of Place in Global Health

Arguably anthropology's sophisticated approach to place is one of its most unique and enduring contributions to the study of global health. As an empirically driven discipline based on extended fieldwork, anthropological approaches to place tend to link history and political economy with detailed ethnographic accounts of everyday lives. While this book is an outcome of my long-term field engagement in Sololá, using the previously mentioned criteria, I do not attempt to treat Sololá or Guatemala as a place. In fact, I do not consider this book to be *about* Sololá in particular or Guatemala more generally. The metaphor of a play is useful for describing the role of Sololá (and Guatemala) in this book, as it serves as a backdrop or stage that is ever present as we consider the protagonists' actions.[18] Yet that backdrop lacks the full depth and complexity of a real place. I refer to these backdrop-like scenes as "ideas of place."

I find myself in a situation similar to that of the anthropologist James Ferguson (2006), who argues that privileging what I might call disciplinarily rigorous approaches to place could be unintentionally obstructionist. Ferguson calls out anthropologists' objection or refusal to engage in conversations about "Africa" as an imagined whole. Ferguson agrees with anthropological scholarship that rebuffs "Africa" and similarly concurs that such depictions were not only unrigorous but potentially deleterious. Yet, in the introduction to his book *Global Shadows: Africa in the Neoliberal World Order*, Ferguson tells the reader that he was moved to take "Africa" seriously after reading yet another *New York Times* article about "Africa." Ferguson argues that "Africa," no matter how empirically unrigorous an imaginary, was exactly the place that was at play in geopolitics. In other words, what was occurring on the ground was frequently motivated and justified by this idea of "Africa." Ferguson contends that anthropological refusal to engage "Africa" not only sidelined anthropological analysis but had the tangible consequence of allowing logics of intervention in "Africa" to go unimpeded.[19]

My research into the domain of global health has undoubtedly led me to the conclusion that global health can be similarly animated by places like Ferguson's "Africa," which are more ideas of places than actual locations. Indeed, anthropologically rigorous treatments of place point out how many global health interventions and programs get place wrong or do not consider it at all. This is an incredibly important anthropological intervention. My own work on the Safe Motherhood Initiative has examined the fallout of an implementation of a set of interventions that were developed in the upper echelons of the WHO and simultaneously implemented on three continents (Berry, 2006, 2008a, 2008b, 2010). Yet, as the medical anthropologist Rob Lorway (2017) argues, many of the main constructs important to operationalizing global health programming and interventions in the formal sector today are predicated on perfecting modes of engagement that intend to supersede context.[20]

The global health scholar Nora Kenworthy and the anthropologist Richard Parker's (2014) description of the global fight to extend antiretroviral therapies (ARVs) provides a concrete example of how modes of global health engagement can shift attention away from context. It notes how the focus on "scaling up," which refers to a policy of dramatically increasing programming to deliver ARVs across a number of sub-Saharan African countries, organized efforts around "a predominantly technocratic shuttling of drugs into bodies," so that "attention to the broader social conditions of HIV infection and the survival of those already infected" was lost (Kenworthy & Parker, 2014:1). Likewise, the anthropologist Vincanne Adams (2013a:84), in unpacking her own experience with evidence-based global public health, reminds us that, when particular standards of practice are centered, "some things are erased." Ethnography is perhaps uniquely equipped to demonstrate that context is more than just a problem—that a lack of understanding of context can lead interventionists and scholars to fallacious conclusions. Furthermore, ethnographies suggest the importance of solutions that arise from particular times in particularly places, letting go of the idea that the value of a solution is related to its ability to be scaled up.

Nevertheless, I agree with Ferguson that we have something to lose when our necessary mode of response to ideas of places is to use our work to reveal its limits or what it "erases." Yet, like "Africa" and other ideas of place, technologies that drive and characterize global health can be generative. For example, Adams (2016) points out that "metrics" (another technology) create an order that enfranchises an increasing fusion between "making money" and global health. Similarly, I have found that ideas of place were important to understand how volunteers engaged with short-term medical missions, as well as how they understood possibility, ambiguity, and risk. Most obviously, short-term medical missions purportedly happen in places where care providers are needed to fill a gap. The volunteers I engaged ended up in Sololá, but typically neither Guatemala nor Sololá itself was central to what they were doing—they could have gone anywhere. Ideas of place, I argue, have become increasingly central to understanding the care regimes being built around patients in low-income settings.

For the most part, Guatemala and Sololá function as ideas of place in these pages because this is an ethnography primarily about people who come to Guatemala. The relationship between global health work and ethical lives is explored in this book almost wholly through North American volunteers' experiences and perspectives. I therefore find it imperative to work from the ideas of place that they articulate, no matter how untethered these ideas might be from the realities of context or how tethered they might be to "medical imaginaries" (Wendland, 2012).

My choice to write an ethnography that does not try to push back against Guatemala as an idea of a place was, nonetheless, difficult. I recognize that this approach threatens to strengthen stereotypes about Guatemala among my readers, further reinscribing power relationships that stem from and underlie myriad inequities, and this causes me discomfort. Notably, a rich body of social science scholarship already exists documenting systemic and structural inequities present in Guatemala, as well as how these inequities impact health and attempts to improve health (Beck, 2017; Berry, 2010; Chary et al., 2013; Grech, 2015; Maupin, 2009; Rasch, 2012; Rohloff, Díaz, & Dasgupta, 2011; Yates-Doerr, 2015). Adopting a narrative structure that purports to position Guatemala and Guatemalans as equal actors would necessarily create a different book with different goals. I have found that writing an ethnography of global health practice that takes seriously these ideas of place and imaginings about self (no matter how empirically untrue) is central to explaining why we see a boom in DIY global health activity, like STMMs. It is also central to understanding how such practices thrive despite the uncertainty that global health volunteers face in the field and the potential for doing harm (Hall-Clifford & Cook-Deegan, 2019).

In making this decision, I have included relevant information about Guatemala in places where protagonists encounter it. Notably, the importance of Guatemala as a setting is most prominent for me (not my interlocutors), as my years spent there frequently shaped my perspective.

## Chapter Outline

Chapter 1 asks how North America volunteers have come to view short-term medical missions as a favored global health opportunity. I build on traditions of anthropologists who remind us that things that seem real, such as globalization (Tsing, 2005), market capitalism (Ho, 2005), and even global health itself (Brada, 2016, 2023), are actually constructed. The chapter considers three major transformations that have occurred over the past two decades that have made STMMs available and appealing to volunteers: an expansion of players in the global health domain to include clinicians; a delinking of global health from the practices that came before it; and the rise of DIY global health. These transformations have made STMMs legible to North Americans as secular and professional global health action. Chapter 1 leaves us open to considering what sort of world this global health action might be building.

Chapter 2 argues that STMMs are not only secular, professional work but important parts of volunteers' ethical lives. I support my contention by drawing on Keane's (2014a, 2016) construct of ethical affordances (or triggers that spark or connect to people's ethical sensibilities) to consider volunteers' ethical reflexivity. I show how the value of STMMs in building volunteers' ethical lives is profoundly personal, derived from sensibilities toward kin and personal understandings of race. Simultaneously, this inquiry opens a deeper exploration of the forces that shape global health action and, thereby, the global health domain itself. The dominant narrative emphasizing a volunteer's desire to help obscures as much about global health action as it reveals—making something nuanced and complicated appear simple and foregone. Shifting our focus to the integration of professional, personal, and ethical lives also sheds doubt on the likelihood that critical scholars' arguments about lack of effectiveness of global health action could impact the scores of people drawn to DIY global health every year.

Within the larger narrative of the book, chapters 1 and 2 help explain volunteers' participation in short-term medical missions as part of both their professional and their ethical lives. These points become critical to subsequent chapters and help us understand how volunteers are making sense of the events that constitute day-to-day life at a medical mission.

Chapter 3 focuses on my personal experiences of volunteering in jornadas, tracing how a few, spectacular moments changed me and thereby reworked my understanding of the relationship between ethical action and STMMs. I consider how my own gut feelings regarding the goodness of my jornada work spoke back to my less positive scholarly analysis of jornada work, leading me to explore visceral ethics. I describe what it was like to be at a jornada to help explain why it generates such strong feelings of having done good.

Chapters 4 and 5 work together to consider the role of visceral ethics in volunteers' judgments of their individual actions as being morally good or creating harms that go against their reasons for being at a jornada. Chapter 4 focuses on the experience of one volunteer across decades to explore the importance of context to making situated judgments of one's own actions. This exploration demonstrates how short-term engagements actually limit the ability of volunteers to understand the effects of their actions on the world. Ultimately, chapter 5 focuses on one clinical encounter to better describe the indeterminacy or uncertainty that frequently characterizes global health work. Taken together, these two chapters argue that volunteers lack the information they need for situated judgments and illustrates why they rely on visceral ethics to understand their ethical actions.

In the conclusion, I review and synthesize my argument that affect plays a generative role in contemporary global health. The importance of affect to global health action is concerning. As we see with visceral ethics, a knock-on effect of affect is that we are soothed into believing that our actions are good and therefore disregard the due diligence necessary to be certain of this. Obviously, if there was no indication that STMMs could be harmful, then there would be no problem. However, when we take a step back to consider how STMMs might be causing unintentional harms, the optimism, I would argue, is unfounded. Luz's story from the prologue demonstrates how good intentions do not necessarily translate into good outcomes. Anthropologists of global health have important insight into the ways that global health interventions (particularly those considered technical and apolitical by their implementers) can produce unintended harms at multiple different levels. Nevertheless, as I argue in the conclusion, rebuffing volunteers' intention to do good only through inquiry into the outcomes of those intentions is missing an important part of the story. Rather, we must learn from how we teach and strive to meet people who want to take global health action "where they are." Global health work is central to many North American's visions of how to live a good life. We need to ask difficult questions that can help people decide if DIY global health opportunities reflect the values they associate with ethical action.

1

# Transformations in Global Health

*Short-Term Medical Missions and Their Appeal to North American Clinicians*

Thirty years ago, a North American physician temporarily working in a clinic in a low- or low-middle-income country (LMIC) would not have been identified as engaging in global health.[1] One of my participants succinctly addressed this when he explained how he had come to work in Guatemala with a short-term medical mission. Simon, who was nearing the end of a successful career working and teaching medicine in elite institutions in the United States, described how in the 1970s he decided to pursue an international medical experience as part of his degree. Simon told me that at that time there was no framework in US medical schools to understand or support what he wanted to do and therefore no institutional support for seeking an international medical elective. Instead, he had to arrange his placement himself by finding and contacting a potential clinic in Guatemala by "snail mail." He found his first placement at the Behrhorst clinic in Guatemala.[2]

Simon's experience at the Behrhorst clinic made such an impression on him that after he returned to the United States and finished medical school, he continued to prioritize his work in Guatemala. Though he completed a few clinical stints in other countries, he always came back. When I interviewed him, he was working in Guatemala at least a couple of weeks a year, frequently through STMMs or other short-term clinical placements. Simon remarked that, despite going to Guatemala consistently since medical school, over the decades, his colleagues have changed how they relate to his international activities as a physician. At first, no one understood or was interested in his work abroad. Now his colleagues easily recognized and labeled what he does as "global health" work.

As Simon's story demonstrates, before contemporary short-term medical missions were a thing, some North Americans found ways to engage in clinical work in LMICs, including Guatemala. Simon described his early work as "tropical medicine," a medical subspeciality (like dermatology or internal medicine) that arose during the colonial era (Greene et al., 2013). Others might have found their way there through religious work. Still others might have participated in medical humanitarianism (which has tended to be distinguished by its response to acute needs like disasters or wars (Abramowitz & Panter-Brick, 2015). Yet Simon's story illustrates that this sort of clinical activity was not common or easily legible to colleagues as pertaining to some domain outside of medicine. Moreover, as I describe shortly, it did not fit into how people at the time thought about activities done under the closest ancestor of global health, which until the end of the 1990s was referred to as "international health."

This chapter addresses an important question: How did short-term medical missions became a popular form of global health work attractive to North Americans? To answer this question, I trace transformations in global health represented by Simon's story that have created spaces where new kinds of actors can participate in DIY activities, like STMMs, outside the confines of traditional structures and ideologies that dominated this domain. Three transformations characterizing global health are important to my explanation. First is a novel integration of clinical (medical) practice into global health, a major diversion from common practice under global health's predecessor, international health. Second is a delinking of global health activity from the historical past. I contrast Christian medical missionaries who played an important role in the colonial era with contemporary STMMs to demonstrate how present-day volunteers envision professional medical missions as unrelated to those that preceded them. I argue that this delinking from the historical past is central to volunteers perceiving global health as an aspect of their own ethical lives. These transformations have underwritten a third: the creation of a robust, informal DIY global health sector, which includes short-term medical missions. Scholars and dominant global health players and practitioners have ignored the informal, DIY global health sector in favor of formal, global health endeavors. As we will see throughout this book, discounting DIY global health has consequences for how we define, teach, and engage global health—consequences that currently undercut attempts to promote health equity.

## From International Health to Global Health: Including Clinical Practice

While activity referred to as "global health" is now so extensive that global health tends to be seen as its own domain, from the 1950s to the1990s, "international health," global health's predecessor, was viewed as a subcomponent of the domain of social and economic development. Development has been strongly influenced by the post–World War II environment (Birn, 2009; Keshavjee, 2014). The word "international" obscures the power relations inherent to the field, which were centered on health programming and interventions done *outside* the borders of high-income countries (HIC), that is, in places we now refer to as LMICs. From the 1960s onward, international health became one of the modes through which geopolitical competition was waged between the United States and the Soviet Union, both aiming to use health interventions to spread influence in former colonies.

Countries and international organizations held a preeminent role in directing international health activity, as most development aid, including that marked for health, was channeled through national institutions like the United States Agency for International Development (USAID), or organizations under the United Nations (UN) umbrella. Most of these international health activities were funded through individual HIC countries giving aid directly to a LMIC that they wanted to influence (i.e., country-to-country giving). Former colonial powers like the United Kingdom and France also depended on international organizations, such as the World Health Organization, to spread their influence. At an operational level, these funding and geopolitical arrangements meant that the everyday work of international health was conducted predominantly by a cadre of professional experts who operated in conjunction with, or for, the public sector (Escobar, 1988, 1995).[3]

Under international health, ministries of health worldwide and international organizations, such as the WHO, dominated clinical practice and thus physician participation. Working as a physician in international health was more of a career choice and less of a gig. Physicians were needed to create strategies and oversee international initiatives and programming, such as WHO's Primary Health Care initiative (Birn & Krementsov, 2018) or UNICEF's Child Survival campaign (Justice,

2000), as well as liaise with ministries of health. They were not needed to do clinical placements or directly care for patients. Indeed, sending a doctor to a clinic was not a strategy that would aid one country's attempt to influence other countries or to exert ideological control.[4] Thus, physicians doctoring in clinics, like Simon with the Berhorst clinic, just did not jibe with international health.

Theodore Brown, Marcos Cueto, and Elizabeth Fee (2006) argue the international debt crisis, which raged through LMICs in the 1980s, began the changes that eventually made Simon's practice legible to his colleagues as "global health." The debt crisis promulgated a shift in Western agendas away from garnering influence by funding development activities (i.e., international health) and toward ensuring that LMICs remained solvent to service their debt.[5] HICs, most prominently the US, pursued this end through the World Bank and International Monetary Fund (IMF) by imposing fiscal austerity measures in the form of structural adjustment programs in LMICs. The loan conditionalities that international financial institutions, like the IMF, imposed on countries through structural adjustment required LMIC governments to reduce public-sector spending (including health), slash government employees' salaries, freeze hiring, remove government subsidies and price controls (including on food staples on which many poorer citizens depended), devalue the national currency (thus making everything more expensive), sell state-owned businesses (such as public companies providing water and electricity), reduce taxes on foreign goods, and weaken government regulations on labor and environment. In theory, structural adjustment programs were meant to correct inefficient economies resulting from too much government interference, promote market-driven solutions to LMIC countries' challenges, and make countries favorable places for private investment to stimulate economic growth. Yet as the physician and anthropologist Salmaan Keshavjee (2014) documents, reality deviated from theory. LMIC governments and citizens frequently despised structural adjustment programs as they exacerbated poverty and inequities.[6] In the health domain, the imposition of such measures routinely resulted in shrinking health-sector funding, frozen salaries and restrictions on hiring in ministries of health, the deterioration of infrastructure, and the predictable absence of needed resources, including medications, to address citizens' health issues (Pfeiffer and Chapman, 2010). Austerity measures thus crippled already-strained ministry-governed health systems in LMICs, eroding the health of countries' most neglected and disenfranchised peoples (Lugalla, 1995). The transfer of HIC governments' attention toward economic solvency of LMICs governments meant that they paid little attention to mitigating poverty and improving health of LMIC populations.[7] Promoting health and wealth was no longer a development priority.

The debt crisis therefore created a vacuum in LMIC health sectors in the 1990s, which eventually began to be filled by what we now call "global health." The first players to attempt to fill this vacuum were nongovernmental organizations; from the 1990s onward, the number of NGOs involved in health work in LMICs skyrocketed (Banks & Hulme, 2012; Mussa et al., 2013; Turshen, 1999).[8] Some of the gaps created by the hiring freeze in public sectors were also filled by citizen volunteers—free labor picked up responsibilities previously held by the state (Muehlebach, 2012; Ossome, 2015). Austerity also led to increases in private-sector funding and activity—bringing business logics into what had previously been the purview of the state. A bevy of new actors including pharmaceutical companies, universities, and philanthropic organizations moved into the space (Szlezák et al., 2010), forming new health initiatives, public-private partnerships, and modes of engagement (Brown, 2015; Crane, 2010; Mahat, Citrin, & Bista, 2018; Samsky, 2012; Storeng & Béhague, 2016). These new actors marked an expansion of global interest in health activities, as well as a massive increase in money available to support health initiatives that aligned with funders' interests. Nirmala Ravishankar et al.'s (2009) novel tracking of development assistance for health demonstrated fourfold growth in funding between the end of the Cold War in 1991 (when HIC governments and the UN were the main funders of health initiatives) and 2007 (when new players and new funders had moved into the space).[9] The term "global health" was increasingly used to describe all of this activity.[10]

Now paltry LMIC government health budgets combined with the explosion of earmarked funding from donors to enfranchise new health initiatives. Rather than pursuing comprehensive primary care through established health systems, programming tended to invest in specific target diseases (such as HIV, TB, or malaria) or health outcomes (such as maternal mortality), an approach referred to as "vertical interventions."[11] Patients who were fortunate enough to have the ailments or to be part of populations that donors were targeting could frequently access high-quality care. Patients whose ailments or identities did not fit within those narrow parameters continued to encounter extraordinary scarcity and difficulty accessing meaningful care (Keshavjee, 2014; McKay, 2017; Nguyen, 2010; Pfeiffer, Montoya, et al., 2010; Street, 2014; Sullivan, 2011). Furthermore, an additional requirement of austerity was freezing salaries and prohibiting the hiring of new staff in the public system. Yet donor-funded, vertical initiatives had access to significant funding, enabling clinics running their programs to offer excellent salaries and better working conditions for health care workers. The result was substantial brain drain from the public system into donor-funded, vertical initiatives (Høg, 2014; Qureshi, 2014). Public clinics and hospitals were encouraged to seek their own sources of funding by imposing user fees that frequently left the poorest without care (Foley, 2010; Lugalla, 1995) or by courting their own donors or by starting side businesses (Marten & Sullivan, 2020). However, working with multiple donors created its own pressures on LMICs' health workers, who were now saddled with collecting data and reporting on a dizzying array of indictors dictated by their donors. All of this work undermined the quality of services that health care workers could deliver in the public system. By the middle of the first decade of this century, all key players, including international organizations, financial institutions, NGOs, and LMIC governments, recognized how austerity measures combined with vertical programs had deteriorated already-weak LMIC health systems (Hafner & Shiffman, 2012; Mishra, 2014; Pfeiffer, Montoya, et al., 2017). In 2007, the WHO published a report arguing that all players were responsible for ensuring that their initiatives strengthened health systems (World Health Organization, 2007), and positive impacts of engagements on LMIC health systems became a priority (Adam & de Savigny, 2012; Hafner & Shiffman, 2012; Pfeiffer & Nichter, 2008; Storeng, 2014; Storeng, Prince, & Mishra, 2018).

By the end of the first decade of this century, the term "global health" was being thrown around to simultaneously describe the players, values, and purposes characteristic of promoting health in LMICs. Many scholars and practitioners engaged or interested in this work found clarity in Jeffrey P. Koplan et al.'s (2009) now-canonical attempt to define "global health" as a new domain.[12] In an article published in the prestigious medical journal *The Lancet*, the authors juxtapose global health with both public health and international health to highlight overlaps and to signal important differences between the domains. Koplan et al. (2009) characterize international health as emphasizing country-to-country aid, usually a former colonial power aiding a former colony. They also point out that international health relied on a restricted core of specialists who were involved in development activities. Global health, by contrast, is characterized by pursuits crossing national and disciplinary boundaries. It replaces the country-to-country aid model with collaborations led by a plethora of new actors—including universities and clinical practitioners. Global health recognizes something that the Ebola epidemic and the COVID-19 pandemic have since taught the broader world: what happens in Freetown, Liberia, or Wuhan, China, can affect Dallas, United States, or Vancouver, Canada. Pursuing health is not just about garnering influence over allies, but rather, health, and the things that threaten it, bind us all together.

Simon's story of doing periodic clinical work in Guatemala is instructive because it points to an important outcome of this transformation from international health to global health. Decades ago, the development or aid world was not organized in a way that a clinician like Simon would be recognized as contributing to international health. Global health, however, is marked by an expansion of players and has created new spaces in which clinicians can imagine themselves participating. While international health was steeped in geopolitics and diplomacy, global health can be characterized by an unfettered mobilization of skill.[13] Suddenly, almost anyone with the time and the resources can find a clinical space from which to "do" global health, including short-term medical missions.

## Delinking Global Health from History: STMMs as Secular, Professional Endeavors

In addition to opening new spaces for clinician participation, working in the global health domain is far more attractive to your average clinician than international health ever would have been. As noted earlier, international health has been characterized by wealthy (former colonial) powers giving money to poor former colonies to garner influence by helping to improve the population's health. Global health, however, is represented as being free from the inequitable power relations that mired international health (Birn, 2009).[14] Koplan et al. point to this transformation as a key feature of the new domain: "The preference for use of the term global health where international health might previously have been used runs parallel to a shift in philosophy and attitude that emphasises the mutuality of real partnership, a pooling of experience and knowledge, and a two-way flow between developed and developing countries" (2009:1994–1995). Global health emphasizes "global cooperation" and "health equity among all nations for all people," rather than HICs "help[ing] people of other nations" (Koplan et al., 2009:1994). In global health, we are now all seemingly working together in partnership for everyone's benefit.

Short-term medical missions are a fascinating place to look at the way current activities in the global health domain become delinked from troubling pasts, enabling a new righteousness in what is now glossed as global health work. Notably, medical missions have an even longer, and somewhat more troubling, history than international health. Medical missions are linked to histories of colonization and more particularly to the hierarchies and power relationships that evolved as part of colonial systems (Jobson, 2018; Nelson, 1999). Religious missionaries—first Catholic in the Spanish and Portuguese empires and, by the nineteenth century, increasingly Protestant, especially in Africa and Asia—reached deep into rural areas, where they scrutinized local practices and cultures and sought to inculcate Christian values, including through medicine (Greene et al., 2013).[15] The historian Megan Vaughan (1991) points out that medical missionaries typically operated on different planes from colonial medical officials. Colonial medical officials' priorities were controlling epidemics in ports and towns and improving worker productivity in zones rich in natural resources (Ngalamulume, 2004). For medical missionaries, who served as key points of contact with, and gathered information about, local populations, the moral "uplift" (Vaughan, 1991:7) of the colonizing process took place one body and soul at a time. Relations between colonial and missionary medics were often marked by suspicion and distrust but also collaboration and mutual dependence, especially after 1900. Missionaries raised funds through their mother churches in Europe and North America, which enabled them to build extensive networks of leprosaria and hospitals (many of which still exist), in which charity and medical and religious proselytization were intertwined, offering a humanitarian rationale for colonialism's so-called civilizing mission (Vongsathorn, 2012).

Histories written about mission work often emphasize relationships between missionaries, colonialism, and the saving of souls (Hardiman, 2006). And indeed, these linkages came up when I interviewed Ralph, a North American clinician who was deeply involved in a health-related NGOs in Guatemala but who, notably, rejected participating in jornadas. When asked what he thought about STMMs, he immediately used language to align short-term medical missions with a colonial past. He critiqued them as "harken[ing] back to the misapprehension of the lore of the safari doctor, tropical cline, quinine quaffing, pith helmet wearing." The poetry of Ralph's quote lies in his evocative description of a colonial doctor. Quinine, a drug from South America, was the main protection from malaria, one of the scourges of the "tropics" that had threatened colonization. Quinine spread through empires most popularly in the form of tonic water, which colonists would commonly mix with alcohol, making the so-called civilized practice of drinking alcoholic cocktails into an ostensible act of responsibility and imbibing, or "quaffing," as self-protection (Barnett, 2012). The evocation of a "quinine quaffing" doctor wearing a "pith helmet" instantly reminds us of times and practices long past. Using the safari doctor to characterize short-term medical missions inherently creates a tension between the past and the present. Indeed, Ralph's words insinuate that the short-term medical mission volunteer is an anachronism, enacting colonial practices that have long since been condemned.[16]

Yet despite these well-documented historical linkages, people working with jornadas did not bring up or reflect on colonial missionaries to define their own work. Moreover, despite the fact that other research has linked Christianity and STMMs (Lasker, 2016), my questions about the role of religion in medical missions never went anywhere. Not one interviewee considered their jornadas as religious; they saw jornadas as connected to their professional identities.

To be sure, many of the interviewees with whom I spoke identified with an organized religion and attended church. On one mission I accompanied, a pastor offered a voluntary nondenominational Christian service every morning before the mission started. Moreover, churches were instrumental in mobilizing economic support for missions. Many volunteers' and organizers' first connections with short-term medical mission work were through their congregations. Churches frequently sponsored and organized medical missions, or individual medical missioners found an STMM in Guatemala through their congregation's recommendations.[17]

Philippe's experience with evangelical medical missions in Sololá illuminates why, despite maintaining connections to churches and holding religious sentiments, jornada volunteers all considered their STMM work as wholly secular, unrelated to past or present religious missions. Philippe and his wife were on vacation in Sololá when he met an evangelical couple from North America staying at their hotel. The couple had just completed a medical mission, and they inspired Philippe with their recounting. As the couples got to know each other, the evangelicals asked Philippe, who was a physician, if he would "feel comfortable doing a medical mission with [them]." Philippe was excited about the prospect and gave the couple his contact information. A few months later, they wrote asking him if he could step in to "save" a planned mission trip.[18] Three nurses and a doctor had been scheduled to go, but the doctor had canceled at the last minute. Philippe "called [his wife] over [and] said, 'Read this. I'm going to Guatemala [laughs] . . . again.'"

Philippe enjoyed his mission work in Sololá so much that he started going three times a year, but all of that came to an end when his wife had an opportunity to accompany the evangelical mission as a translator. Translation put her in a different part of the mission's organizational flow, and she quickly realized that medicine was not the only goal. She relayed to Philippe that the organizers running the mission made converting to the evangelical form of Christianity that they followed a precondition of seeing the doctor. Those who did not want to become evangelical were turned away. Neither Philippe nor his wife thought that it was acceptable to deny a person medical treatment based on their faith or to strongarm someone into changing their faith to access treatment. They never accompanied this evangelical organization on a mission again.

Philippe's description of an evangelical medical mission as one that "had an agenda to save people in other ways"—by which he meant trying to save souls—fit well with how volunteer interviewees thought about the difference between secular, professional missions that they worked with and evangelical missions. Interviewees' claim that missions were secular was a disavowal of what Philippe refers to as "other ways" to help, as well as a statement about medical assistance being the dominant and only priority in STMMs. No one I interviewed was comfortable with the idea of evangelizing during a medical mission.

Volunteers also argued that allowing evangelical interests to dominate medical interests minimized the quality of patient care in missions. Typically, in an evangelical medical mission, any medical professional who was a congregant and willing to travel would form a team. Secular missions, on the other hand, usually recruited personnel with an eye toward the type of services that they wanted to offer.[19] Thus, interviewees felt that an evangelical mission's ability to meet patients' needs was coincidental, rather than deliberate. Furthermore, evangelical medical missions were rumored to include retired and now unlicensed practitioners, thus allowing individuals who could not practice medicine in North America to practice in Guatemala. They prioritized religious salvation over medical regulation. My participants considered both practices transgressive and unethical. Whether or not participants identified with any religion, to them, short-term medical missions should employ licensed professionals to work on bodies, not save souls.

Ana's case provides an excellent example of how short-term medical mission volunteers prioritize their identities as medical professionals participating in global health action, regardless of their individual religious affiliation. Ana was a veteran mission surgeon and a self-identifying churchgoing Catholic. Before participating in the jornada where I encountered her, she had volunteered at another mission organized by a Catholic diocese in another Latin American country, where the patients were treated in a Catholic hospital. When Ana described the mission, she said, "It's a religious-affiliated mission, but it's very secular in terms of the work that gets done." Most of the patients were Catholic and, as she said, "would probably love it [if we prayed for them] because they're very religious." The sister who organized the mission offered a voluntary scripture reading every morning. But there was no praying, no talking about religion, and, she emphasized, any medical personnel, including atheists, were welcome to join. The focus was on medicine.

Ana discussed her views of missions and religion, saying, "I don't consider it part of religious work. I consider it part of just being good to each other, which is in alignment with being Christian, but it's not—that's not why I'm there. . . . As the practical human being that I am, and as somebody who believes in a higher power, I would much rather go over there and fix your cleft palate and take out your cataract than go do Bible study. If you're going to spend the money, spend the resources, get your team together. . . . I'm much more practical about that." Ana's statement made it clear that she wore her medical hat on these missions. For her, missions were about going "over there" and "fix[ing]" the problem. She differentiated this mission from a trip organized around "Bible study." In her last sentence, Ana made it clear that "Bible study" was not a sufficient activity to warrant the "money" and "resources" that it took for volunteers to travel. Ana emphasized that, for her, it was just "practical" to need to see a tangible "fix" as a return for volunteers putting so many resources into arranging and paying for a trip. In short, a "Bible study" trip was not cost-effective.

Stephanie's case offers another perspective of how a decidedly religious person leveraged her professional, medical identity to explain her work in STMMs. Stephanie viewed her ability to travel and practice medicine as a gift from God. She said, "I feel like [God] gave me skills as a [medical specialist] to go and help people. Even though I wasn't down there talking about religion, I was okay with that, because I was providing the services and the gifts that I've been given to help other people." Though Stephanie was receptive to participating in a religious-based mission where the goal would be, in Ana's words, "Bible study," Stephanie was definitive about the fact that a medical mission must prioritize biomedical care. When asked about the role of religion in medical missions, Stephanie judged the idea of triaging people for their religious beliefs as unacceptable. She said, "Being selective about who gets to receive medical care, . . . that doesn't seem right to me. I feel like if we're going to help people, we're going to help people." Stephanie's statement communicates her belief that medical missions are about medical work. Her elision of the ideas of "help" and "receiving medical care" leaves no room for competing agendas. She later clarified this point more directly when she stated, "I just think that we're there to help people from a medical standpoint. I just think that that's the bigger goal, the bigger picture."

Ashley, who worked through her church and congregation to organize missions with a partner church in Sololá, further argued that religious goals were inappropriate for any short-term missions, including medical ones. She framed her point by describing to me the "disaster" that was one religious mission: "One of the worst things I've ever seen on an airplane going down was the team that all had matching T-shirts with the slogan, 'Bringing God to Guatemala.'" From her perspective, this mission not only denigrated the resources available in Guatemala by assuming that God was not there and that volunteers had to "bring God" but also supported the idea that these volunteers' action alone could easily transform the world. Ashley was adamant that her volunteers think differently. She explained to me how short-term medical missions could be about "living our faith" through medical work but not by talking to people about God. Through her years of working on missions, Ashley had a clear idea of the limits of the type of work that could be accomplished in the short term. She told me, "I explain to my group, our job is not to go down and try to, in one week's time, create a faith community with people with whom we can communicate at a very elementary level, at best, and will not be there to establish it." The focus of the trip was to work alongside people in Guatemala and provide extra resources to buttress what already existed. Ashley's groups accomplished this by making sure that churches supported the development of medical capacity in communities and that medical volunteers from North America worked alongside local people to build their skills.

Perhaps because Ashley relied on her faith as a major resource for organizing and funding mission work, she found herself needing to defend her insistence on a separation between professional and religious work to mission volunteers and supporters. She recounted one specific incident: "Last year, there was a young woman from the Baptist church who came with us, and she asked me that question. She said, 'What good does it do to heal their bodies if we're not doing anything for their souls?' I had that conversation with her that our part of that is trying to provide an environment where health can flourish so that those who carry out that ministry there don't have to—can begin that work at a place with healthy bodies." This exchange illustrates how volunteers calibrate their mission involvement to their religious identities, while prioritizing their STMMs as part of a professional, global health domain. In Ashley's assessment, the spiritual life of Guatemalans who attend jornadas was not irrelevant; rather, spirituality could not be adequately or responsibly addressed through the short-term medical mission model. What she believed could be addressed through this model was improving individuals' health. As she saw it, volunteers in Guatemala aimed to provide medical care to help create "healthy bodies."

Ashley's contention that you can separate working for "healthy bodies" from saving "souls" stakes out how participants separate the short-term medical missions they were involved with from missions in the past and from evangelical missions of the present. The preceding narratives also help characterize medical missions as professional work in the global health domain.[20] Participants and organizers spoke about short-term medical missions as a contemporary practice devoted to improving health outcomes. Even participants who felt that volunteering for a jornada was inspired by, or fulfilling, God's plan for them were clear in seeing mission work as clinical, global health work.

Despite the clear distinctions participants draw between short-term medical mission work and colonial missions work, comparing my research with the anthropologist Britt Halvorson's study of volunteers in religious medical-aid organizations reveals STMM volunteers' relative lack of concern with the past. Halvorson conducted multiyear research with two different Lutheran NGOs in Minnesota that had decades-old, direct partnerships with churches in Madagascar. Halvorson's (2018:3) contemporary volunteers maintained a palpable awareness of the potentially fraught connections between their own work and their predecessors' missionary work, which was characterized by colonialism and "cultural imperialism of colonial evangelism." Like my own approach in this chapter, Halvorson focuses on continuities and discontinuities with the history that underwrites the volunteering that she studied. For volunteers to make volunteer work consonant with their ethical lives, Halvorson describes how they define what they do now as "humanitarian work" that is "qualitatively different" from what their predecessors did. For example, they now prioritized sending medical aid over sending Minnesotans to Madagascar in a belief that noninterference mitigates colonial power dynamics produced in past face-to-face missions. One leaves Halvorson's ethnography with a clear view of the continuity of the past to the present and both the remembering and forgetting that volunteers must engage in to change medical aid as a field. Comparing Halvorson's descriptions to my own draws into sharp relief the absence of volunteers' and NGO organizers' preoccupation with aligning or distancing their own work with anything that came before it, shoring up this characterization of global health as delinked from the past.

Delinking of global health from historical antecedents is an important transformation that has further enfranchised STMMs as an appealing activity within the contemporary global health domain. As the global health scholar Anne-Emanuelle Birn (2009) points out, this delinking has effectively distanced global health from many of the critiques that mired international health, resulting in, I contend, a patina of righteousness that makes global health work a natural fit for (North Americans') ethical lives. The delinking has also allowed volunteers to reimagine missions as singularly professional, clinical activities that are unconnected to Christianity (or politics). Volunteers connect STMMs with an opportunity to use their own professions to do the good work that they want to do. I now turn to the third transformation in the global health domain that has enfranchised STMMs: the rise of DIY global health.

## DIY Global Health

My first encounter with a medical mission, which occurred over twenty years ago, provides an instructive example that helps define DIY global health. That medical mission was composed of a group of medical students and instructors from a university in Florida. They traveled to Guatemala with selections of medications and blindly chose locations to visit on a map. Without previous announcement, they arrived at the town I lived in, informed the auxiliary nurse in the health post of their purpose, and began setting up pop-up tents in the central square. Among the medications they brought were anthelmintics—drugs designed to treat infections of parasitic worms. They set up a station to dispense them to school-aged children; in exchange for taking the medication, each child received a candy. I can imagine that if someone were in a room in Florida trying to plan valuable therapeutic actions that supervised medical students could undertake over the course of a day, deworming school-aged children would seem promising.[21] Epidemiologic studies have long documented high rates of helminth infections in Guatemala (Anderson et al., 1993; Lauritz et al., 2009; Sorensen et al., 2011) and suggested that untreated infections can have negative health effects (Taylor-Robinson et al., 2012).

Nonetheless, despite how contradictory it might seem, at the time, you would have been hard-pressed to find anyone who was employed by the Guatemalan Ministry of Health or any of the international organizations that staffed and funded health initiatives who would have thought rolling into a town and dosing children would be helpful, for several reasons. First, it was already being done.[22] The Guatemalan Ministry of Health has worked at the center of intersectoral collaborations to decrease the impacts of parasitic diseases, particularly among children. To this day, part of its effort involves following the WHO blueprint to hold health campaigns (also referred to as jornadas in Guatemala) every six months, where schoolchildren receive drugs to reduce helminth infections (MSPAS, 2022). However, treatment of acute infections is only one part of an effective response (Strunz et al., 2014). The Ministry of Health jornadas also offer preventative education, informing participants (including children) about what helminth infections are, how you get them, and how to work within the confines of current conditions to reduce future infection (e.g., hand washing).[23] Second, this is not a case where more is better. Regarding the safety of anthelmintics, WHO guidelines suggest that populations like schoolchildren in Guatemala, who are in a high-risk category, receive only two doses per year. Even the safest and most used anthelmintics like albendazole have been associated with toxicity-related liver damage (Amoruso et al., 2009; Ben Fredj et al., 2014; Grama et al., 2020; Marin Zuluaga et al., 2013). Soon after the Florida team left, my husband noted that he had watched children run away and then get back in line for another dose, eager for another candy. Later, the director of this health district in Sololá told us that children in the town had received doses of anthelmintics six weeks prior to the Floridian mission through their regular school-based jornada. In sum, the Florida jornada's use of anthelmintics was irresponsible, if not dangerous for children.[24]

I had been working in social and economic development in Latin America on and off for about a decade by the time I met the Florida jornada, and I found it surprising how much the Florida jornada differed from other interventions I had seen. At a moment in history when coordinated action to change health outcomes was the flavor of the day, this jornada was not bound to any other organizations. Not only did it lack a partnership with a relevant government agency in Guatemala, but it did also not have any Guatemalan counterpart—not a school or a church or an NGO. In fact, it had no on-the-ground contacts at all. Despite its pop-up tents and medicine, visually, the jornada did not look like other interventions I had seen, the majority of which were marked by fleets of sport utility vehicles bearing organization or project logos on their doors. The Floridians did not even hang up a banner or leave a poster or brochure. Besides the potential illness that could be caused by the meds they handed out, the Floridians left no footprint.[25]

This ability to create and deliver an intervention according to one's own rules was notable when comparing the Florida jornada to other programs and initiatives. Even in the smallest, most grassroots projects, administrative procedures were considered an important component of due diligence. A small grassroots project had to have purpose, an organizational structure (including an elected leadership team), and documentation of actions. Funding placed constraints shaping what a small organization could do. Attracting funding from a larger organization required you to justify a need for a program, contextualize the program in relation to how other communities or organizations were solving this need, and describe to the funder the outcomes of the program at the end of a funding cycle. And this was just small-scale work. Midscale organizations, like many NGOs, and large-scale health interventions undertaken by international and country-to-country aid organizations were necessarily enmeshed into networks, global development initiatives, and government partnerships. These entanglements created constant dialogue and feedback that shaped as well as constrained programs. In short, there was no domain—not civil society, not international health, not humanitarian relief or religious organizations (which tended to involve church partnerships)—where you could do a health intervention with no leadership, connection to context, or accountability to place. For these reasons, what the Florida jornada was doing was worthy of note.

The Florida jornada provides an excellent heuristic (an aid to learning) that draws attention to some of the core characteristics common to DIY global health but uncommon outside of it.[26] DIY global health tends to be self-funded through participant contributions or donations from people in HICs (Fechter & Schwittay, 2019). It can operate on a low budget with little accountability to people, organizations, or the government where DIY global health takes place (Kinsbergen, 2019). As a result, it can set its own goals outside of norms or competing initiatives that might be taking place. With reference to jornadas, we see that this translates into operating on technical, clinical guidelines alone.[27]

DIY global health is also comparatively nimble. For example, one can choose a place to work on a map or by a referral from a friend; if that does not work, DIY global health is flexible enough to move at any point to new opportunities that appear more fertile. It is "ephemeral" (Citrin, 2010). A DIY global health project can exist for as little as three to six months. This core characteristic was also demonstrated in the prologue. That Toronto jornada that treated Luz seemingly produced enduring, written records of its activities (i.e., not ephemeral). Yet once the jornada was over, the organizer no longer held her post, and there was no central location to store (or plans to reference) records. Rather, she put the records in her basement, where they were subsequently lost.

Because DIY global health operates outside of the accountability structures, regulations, and supervision that are inherent to formal global health initiatives, how DIY global health manifests itself is flexible. You can have an intervention, like the Florida jornada, that has all the DIY characteristics. Just as possible are STMMs staffed by medical professionals (like those that I accompanied for this research), which only have a few characteristics of DIY global health. The relative freedom of DIY organizers to tailor and dictate global health action makes DIY global health varied as well as inclusive, creating options to participate in global health that are unfathomable within formal global health activities. Though perhaps DIY global health seems limited to nongovernmental or private voluntary organizations that operate outside of formal global health, we can also see DIY initiatives undertaken by more enduring organizations, including medical schools, that may or may not have links into formal global health activities.

The scant data that we have suggest that DIY global health is a force to be reckoned with. Lasker (2016) estimates that in the United States alone, over two hundred thousand people participate in some form of global health volunteering each year and that citizens' interest in DIY opportunities continues to increase (Fechter & Schwittay, 2019). Nonetheless, professional and scholarly attention remains unduly focused on formal global health efforts, like those attached to established international organizations, philanthropic endeavors, governments, and NGOs.[28] I would argue that DIY global health has been neglected precisely because it does not conform to what many scholars and practitioners in the domain consider important. Specifically, because DIY global health is unpredictable and ephemeral, its on-the-ground influence is limited; it does not influence policy, and it is a disparate set of practices that cannot be systematically scaled up. Yet precisely because it is not typical of formal global health, DIY global health heightens our attention to what is *possible* in the global health domain. This difference is incredibly important to my research because, as the Florida jornada demonstrated, in the absence of regulation, accountability, supervision, and the like, DIY global health creates new possibilities to engage in egregious ways.[29]

## Contemporary Global Health and the Rise of Short-Term Medical Missions

This ethnography is motivated by a central finding: transformations over the past twenty years have paved the way for affect to become a generative force shaping global health. As noted earlier, this finding is important because despite the acknowledgment of the relative importance of affect in adjacent literatures on volunteering or medical humanitarianism, affect has been overlooked as important to global health. Certainly, part of why this story has yet to be told is the relative novelty of the global health domain itself. Perhaps another is that by ignoring the importance of DIY global health in scholarship, we have missed how recent transformations in global health have created a space for affect to be so influential.

I have emphasized three components of contemporary global health (clinical work as global health work, the delinking of global health from past practices, and DIY global health) that are central to the rise of short-term medical missions as a popular form of global health action. The first, growing recognition of clinical work as global health work, has opened avenues of inclusion for clinicians that were not previously available. Concomitantly, the medical field has increasingly come to value global health, as reflected in a preoccupation with how to train students and residents (Drain et al., 2007; Haq et al., 2000; Izadnegahdar et al., 2008; Nelson et al., 2008). STMMs have become an important mode through which any North American clinician (not just those at teaching universities) can participate in this now-valued global health domain. The rise of participation has, in turn, generated a parallel rise in ethical critiques and questions of how to do STMMs better (Asgary & Junck, 2013; Maractho et al., 2022; Prasad et al., 2022).

The second component, a delinking from past practices, has imbued global health with important moral authority; to paraphrase Andrea Cornwall and Karen Brock (2005), it is associated with "good things." Certainly, international health, due to its ties with colonialism and the Cold War, was arguably fraught, if not negative; that stain does not mark global health. The delinking of global health has enabled a new emphasis on cooperation and equitable power dynamics, made more believable by an expanded field of players with innovative modes of engagement. This delinking has created an overwhelmingly positive valence that, as I argue later, has frequently hijacked the motivation of those who work in the domain to ask important questions about its practical impact.[30]

Finally, DIY global health makes it possible for anyone to take global health action free from the constraints typical of formal global health, including partnerships, grant- or contract-based funding, and coordination in host countries (Kinsbergen, 2019). DIY global health means that clinicians can self-organize their own responses, flying under the radar (Fechter & Schwittay, 2019) and remarkably free from outside accountability. For clinicians who may not have the professional bandwidth to join more formal actions within the global health domain, this nimbleness and freedom to practice on their own schedules based on their own goals is incredibly alluring.

While this chapter has established why volunteering in an STMM has become a popular form of global health action available for North Americans, I have only alluded to the connections between STMMs and volunteers' ethical lives. In chapter 2, I draw on my own experiences at STMMs as well as conversations and interviews to attend more specifically to how STMMs engaged volunteers' ethical lives. We will see how performing a professional activity at a jornada can help a volunteer live the type of life they aspire.

2

# Global Health as Profoundly Personal

*Race, Kinship, and Volunteering*

It's a part of just my worldview that I think humans should
help each other.
—Bob, a jornada volunteer, commenting on his global
health work

While most North American volunteers whom I spoke to for this project
had some concerns or suggested improvements for short-term medical
missions, only Alexander, a senior specialist working at a US teaching
hospital, expressed full-on regret. Indeed, when I reached out to him by
email, he was reluctant to set up a time to talk to me. Nevertheless, he
invited me to send him some questions, which I did. I did not expect to
hear from him again, and I was surprised when Alexander wrote back.
While he had not wanted to participate in a congratulatory conversation about STMMs, he responded to me because he found my questions
"serious and analytical." There was no particular negative event that
marred Alexander's experience volunteering for a STMM. In fact, he
made sure to stress the integrity of his fellow volunteers, noting that
he got "a sense of goodwill and self-sacrifice from those around [him],
which are important elements of beneficence." Nevertheless, he regret-
ted participating, as he thought that the jornada he went on was not
intentional enough to help Indigenous people "facilitate their [own]
betterment." He felt that change in Guatemala ultimately needed to be
led by Indigenous people and had imagined that his work there would
provide skills and education that could further this goal. That did not
happen, leading to his feelings that the jornada's activity was useless at
best, damaging at worst. Alexander voiced discomfort at his fellow volunteers' "expressed self-satisfaction with the good that they were doing"
in Sololá.

Alexander's example helps us see how important short-term medical missions are to a volunteer's *ethical* life. More specifically, volunteering at a STMM is action defined by "values and ends that are not in turn defined as the means to some further ends" (Keane, 2016:4). Alexander chose to volunteer at an STMM because he wanted to spend his time and money to help Indigenous people become more independent, and he thought that his volunteering would do this. The vast majority of North Americans I talked to, however, were more like the volunteers Alexander worked with and participated in a jornada to do good for or help others. Indeed, interviewees' responses regarding the ethical imperative to volunteer assumed that people in places that are not the United States or Canada surely need our help and that, by going to those places, we are engaging in meaningful, helpful work.[1]

To better explore STMMs in volunteers' ethical lives, I decided to apply a theoretical frame that situates ethics in relation to participants' actions (instead of what they say) and see what emerged. This approach differs from that of most of my colleagues, who have done a good job of helping us understanding self-reported motivation to volunteer across domains of civic engagement (Eliasoph, 2013), global health engagement (Heron, 2007), and clinical global health travel (Lasker, 2016; Sullivan, 2016). Webb Keane's (2014a) theory of "ethical affordances" was inspirational for directing my analysis of the material that formed this chapter. In my adaptation of Keane's work, ethical affordances are facets of the external world that articulate with or trigger our own reflexivity regarding how we should live or who we should be.[2]

Inspired to see what I could learn by adapting ethical affordances as a theoretical frame, I began by assembling moments during participant observation that stood out as remarkable to me. Some, like the focus of the next section, were interactions that I witnessed. Others were things that people said to me. Many of these moments had already been marked in reflections in my field notes or by memos during my initial data analysis. Once I had this subset of data assembled, I took inspiration from the idea of "ethical affordances" to focus on finding references to things that volunteers perceived as transforming their STMM work from purely medical to both medical and ethical. I found two recurring phenomena that encouraged participation in STMMs by tapping into volunteers' aspirations to live ethical lives: race and kinship.

The medical anthropologist Daisy Deomampo's (2016) ethnography *Transnational Reproduction: Race, Kinship, and Commercial Surrogacy in India* does an excellent job of theoretically situating race and kinship in a way that makes sense for my project on DIY global health. Deomampo insists that we examine North American and European ideologies of kinship and race and how they underwrite transnational practices, of which STMMs are certainly one. For example, Deomampo points out the intertwining of ideologies around "race" and "rescue" that White parents articulate in connection with hiring Indian surrogates to gestate their babies. In this case, narratives emphasize how the White parent paying an Indian (i.e., race) woman contributes to positively changing that Indian woman's life (i.e., rescue). Moving forward, I use Deomampo's theoretical insight into how parents' ideologies of kinship and race embed and reflect existing global dynamics to guide my own analysis.

More specifically, the data I present clearly demonstrate how race and kinship encourage participation in STMMs as part of volunteers' ethical lives. However, Deomampo's insight that volunteers' ideologies around race and kinship are constructed in relation to already-existing global dynamics functions as a missing piece that helps us make sense of a wider context that volunteers leave implicit. Particularly, the global dynamics that volunteers perceive as underwriting STMMs as a transnational practice emphasize the relative privilege of North Americans. Closely following from this is the relative lack of privilege of people living in places where STMMs take place. Of course, there are many dimensions of privilege, but a key one that comes across in these data is the assumption that Guatemalans, and particularly Indigenous Guatemalans, are poor (or poorer) than volunteers. Deriving from this assumption is that providing free medical care at a jornada is an important intervention volunteers undertake to support poor, Indigenous people.

## Race and Ethical Lives: Helping Indigenous People

When examining the corpus of data that I assembled for this chapter, the perceived Indigeneity of patients at jornadas was clearly key to many volunteers' feelings that working at a medical mission was righteous work. This section is crafted around one particular interaction that highlights how "race" emerges as integral to jornada volunteers' feelings that STMM work is action consonant with their own ethical lives. The interaction occurred between a volunteer, whom I will call Matthew, and a patient, Carmen. Matthew was an older physical therapist from the United States who told me that he carved out time every year to serve on a mission, like that in Guatemala. Carmen was a local business owner in a town in Sololá. I was present for this interaction as an English-to-Spanish translator.[3] I begin by reviewing the details of Matthew and Carmen's interaction. I draw on the work of the linguistic anthropologist Nick Enfield (2011) to clarify how we can extract intent and meaning from this interaction. More specifically, examining the interaction helps us establish how Matthew's orientation toward race motivates what he considers to be ethical action—that is, working at a jornada. The anthropologist Clarence Gravlee gives us direction to help make sense of Mathew's perception of Indigeneity as what I am calling race in this chapter (Dressler, Oths, & Gravlee, 2005; Gravlee, 2009; Gravlee & Sweet, 2008; Non & Gravlee, 2015; Tsai et al., 2020). More specifically, Gravlee directs us to consider jornada volunteers' treatment of race as biological as "a worldview."

The events leading to Matthew and Carmen's meeting were set into motion when Carmen missed her footing and fell down some steps at the municipal market. She was in pain and unable to walk comfortably in her high heels, and those who helped her up suggested that she seek help from the medical missioners who were in town. I first encountered Carmen when she sat down on the examining table and told me about her fall and why she had come. After describing the events, Carmen asked if the care was free or if there would be a charge. I translated her question. Matthew said that they would see all Mayan people for free. I translated his response. Carmen stared at me blankly. After a moment, Carmen asked again if there was a charge, so I again translated her question. Matthew affably replied that, as long as you have "the right color skin," then care was free. I told Carmen what Matthew had said. Carmen was flummoxed and silent. Matthew then asked about her injury.

Reviewing this interaction step-by-step can help us better understand what occurred. We hold normative expectations about how any face-to-face interaction ought to unfold. Indeed, Enfield (2011:288) reminds us that Carmen and Matthew's conversation can be viewed as a series of statements that are "hooked together" or that follow from one another (rather than as a series of independent statements). The interaction starts when Carmen asks a question regarding whether she needs to pay for her care. If Carmen asks a question, what follows should approximate an answer to that question. We should read Matthew's response, then, as his answer to Carmen. Matthew answers that all Indigenous people are seen for free. After he answers, in her next turn, Carmen repeats her question. Why would Carmen repeat her question? If she already received an answer, then repeating her question would violate our expectations of standard conversation. At the same time, we expect that when we ask a question, an answer should be forthcoming, and if we fail to get an answer, we are entitled to continue searching. In other words, Carmen is entitled to repeat her question if she considers that Matthew has failed to adequately answer it. Thus, we can assume that she does not feel that Matthew answered her question. Once she repeated herself, Matthew again responded. Yet this time, Matthew modulated his answer to Carmen, mentioning again Indigenous people's right to free care, but this time with reference to Indigenous people's purported skin color.

Enfield's (2011) work entreats us to consider also the conditions under which Matthew's contributions might be interpreted as appropriate or collaborative. Acting as translator and observer to the interaction, I believe that this is reasonable; I saw no evidence that Matthew was intentionally trying to violate conversational expectations or to solicit sanction from or to disrespect Carmen. Indeed, during and after this conversation, Matthew was as affable as ever. Given that nothing was untoward, we expect Matthew to answer Carmen's question; certainly, from Matthew's perspective, he was answering Carmen's question. However, the fact that he continually emphasized that Indigenous people did not need to pay makes sense only if he believed that Carmen was Indigenous. He was saying to Carmen, essentially, "Because you are an Indigenous person, you do not need to pay."

Carmen did not understand Matthew's answers and thus repeated her question because, in Guatemala, Carmen did not present herself as an Indigenous person.[4] Racial hierarchies in the United States are closely tied to the idea that skin color is a good proxy for race and/or ethnicity; ethnic identification in Guatemala is based on numerous factors, including one's personal aesthetic expression and identity allegiance (Hale,

2006; Mendez-Dominguez et al., 1975). For example, Carmen was not wearing a *huipil* or a *corte*, the blouse and skirt typically worn by Indigenous women. Rather, she was wearing a business suit with a tight pencil skirt, a matching jacket and blouse, and high heels. She had short hair and a permanent that added curl. Among Indigenous Mayan communities, feminine adornments involve braiding or weaving cloth into the hair, which is difficult to do with short hair, and longer hair tends to be more common. Carmen was speaking Spanish. While many Indigenous women speak Spanish and some are monolingual Spanish speakers, Spanish is not a traditional language of Indigenous communities in Guatemala. Nonetheless, Carmen's fluency and accent, paired with her appearance (particularly her clothing and hairstyle), indicated that she was probably not Indigenous but rather Ladino, the dominant ethnicity. Even if Carmen had been born to an Indigenous family, her appearance suggested that she did not identify as such now.[5] Carmen repeated her question because she wanted to know about the fee for people who were not Indigenous. Yet, as the interaction progressed, it became clear that Matthew saw her as an Indigenous person.[6]

While a step-by-step review of this interaction might outline what occurred, it does not explain what Matthew is trying "to do" (Austin, 1962)—that is, to achieve or to socially accomplish—with his words. Despite the fact that he was asked an informational question (i.e., "Is the care free, or is there a fee?"), he does not answer (e.g., "Yes, you have to pay," or "No, this is free"). He leaves the domain of the individual clinical encounter between himself and Carmen and instead characterizes his work vis-à-vis "all Mayan people." This statement reveals Matthew's perception of his encounter with Carmen; in essence, he was saying, "My people are here to give to your people." Matthew used his utterance to try to ally himself with Mayan people.

In sum, we can recover the following information from this interaction. Matthew imputed folk concepts that tied human variation to race and then race to biology ("the right skin color"), making race into something innate and, thus, easy for Matthew to identify. Matthew considered people he saw in Guatemala who had "the right skin color" as Indigenous Mayan. Mayan constituted a race different from his own, and this was a key point for Matthew.[7] His comments about free care also highlighted that there was something important about his purportedly different race providing free care to this particular race.[8] Indeed, following Deomampo (2016), placing Matthew's ideology of race, which is active in his transnational practice, in relationship to global dynamics helps explain why he might perceive Indigenous people in Guatemala as generally in need. Moreover, my colleagues' work on relations between biomedicine and race in sub-Saharan African helps flesh out larger and more specific global dynamics that might contribute to why Matthew deems it notable to volunteer among Indigenous people (Crane, 2013; Sullivan, 2018).

As discussed earlier, STMM work is professional, clinical work; yet, as we can see from this interaction, for Matthew, jornada work holds a particular valence for his own ethical life. While Matthew treated Carmen's ankle, he referenced his work in relation to a larger value—that is, free medical treatment for all Mayan people. His perception of the color of Carmen's skin prompted him to reflect on and position his work in this way, reaffirming how his volunteering was simultaneously driven by and realizing his values. The interaction between Matthew and Carmen illustrates how this racial worldview positions race in a way that can galvanize people like Matthew to seek out and volunteer at a jornada.

Matthew was not alone in making Indigenous people central to the ethics of his jornada service. Another notable example occurred when I was outside a compound where a jornada was taking place. For this jornada, I was not a translator per se; rather, I was triaging patients who were waiting in line. I saw a small, four-door car pull up. Two young adults, a middle-aged person and an older woman, got out, and the driver pulled away to park. Later, when I was inside the compound filling out pre-clinic paperwork, I had an opportunity to talk to the family that had pulled up in the car—two grown children, their parents, and their grandmother. The family had been vacationing in a nearby resort town when they heard about the jornada with doctors from North America. They decided to stop on their way back to Guatemala City to see if they could get free medical attention for the grandmother. I then moved on to other patients and did not see that family again. However, during dinner with other volunteers that night, the fact that this family had sought specialist care came up in conversation at my table, and, in trying to specify whom we were talking about, I characterized the family as Ladino, the dominant ethnicity in Guatemala, not Mayan. Phil, one of the physicians I happened to be eating dinner with, was outraged when he heard that the grandmother had been seen. He said that he was there to treat poor, Indigenous people, not people from the capital who were on vacation.[9] We then got into a conversation about the policy of the jornada, which was to treat everyone seeking care. Indeed, working in triage, my job was to document people's ailments, not assess their ethnic or class identity. This policy was a surprise for him. He assumed that we were screening at the door to ensure that only Indigenous people were admitted.

While Phil's remarks were not as direct as Matthew's regarding race, they nonetheless indicate that Phil considered it feasible to screen people for being Indigenous.[10] Like Matthew, Phil implied that there are some empirically recoverable traits that separate Indigenous from non-Indigenous people. Matthew's and Phil's comments point to the idea that there is something durable and external about being Indigenous—like, for example, skin color—that cannot be faked. Matthew and Carmen's misunderstanding illustrated the complexity of the correspondence between purported race and ethnic identity in Guatemala. People signal their identities through various flexible means, including dress, hair style, and language. As Charles R. Hale (2006) points out, someone who identified and presented as Indigenous last year may identify and present as Ladino this year. This complexity complicates Phil's assumption that it would be possible to triage for Indigeneity at the door. Phil's approach echoes Matthew's and points toward what Gravlee (2009) calls a racial "worldview" that conceptualizes Indigeneity as biological and visually recoverable.

For Phil, the idea of serving Indigenous people is closely tied to his valuing the jornada as an important ethical practice. He was affronted that he might have traveled to Guatemala solely to practice medicine for anyone who asked. His belief that he was going to doctor Indigenous people, and particularly poor Indigenous people, was what made this trip worthwhile to him. Like Matthew, Phil was working in a space where I saw a preponderance of Ladinos and many well-off Indigenous families. Unlike me, Phil saw everyone there as Indigenous, and—crucially—doing so was important to him. For this reason, Phil was surprised and offended to learn that a well-off, non-Indigenous family had brought their grandmother to the jornada for medical attention.

These examples portray the importance of race to fomenting the perception that volunteering at a jornada is part of a volunteer's ethical life. Both Matthew and Phil provided medical care back in the United States, probably to a wide variety of patients. Yet, due to assumptions about the race of their patients, they saw care provision in Guatemala as more than just a professional practice. Doctoring Indigenous patients was perceived as bringing a new ethical dimension to their work that differed from their North American practices. Their perceptions of race were important to galvanizing their decision to volunteer for jornadas as well as "center . . . the question of how one should live and what kind of person one should be" (Keane, 2016:20).

## Kinship and Medical Missions

One of the field notes that I had written and that I scrutinized for this chapter involved my surprise at the number of family members who were volunteering together at short-term medical missions. These included parents and children, intergenerational teams of grandparents, parents, and children, and married couples. In this section, I explore how kin relations were taken up by volunteers to connect the importance of jornadas to their ethical lives. Kin relations frequently galvanized ethical reflections, leading volunteers to action. Like race, kin relations also informed and modulated the value of participating in a medical mission, moving it beyond the professional into the ethical.

I was surprised to find so many parent-child teams on missions because I had assumed that professional capacities were a prerequisite for joining short-term medical missions, and in many families, children were not qualified medical professionals. However, larger STMMs needed volunteers who could operate in a support capacity. For example, I generally did things like translating, organizing patients, or starting patient files, but there was a diversity of roles available that anyone could do, including cooking or cleaning, and other roles that could accommodate beginning clinical skills, like assisting pharmacists to put medications in bags or working with nurses in recovery. This structure created the opportunity for missioners with nonmedical skills to travel with their medically skilled family members and provide support for the jornada.

Heather's experience of doing a mission with her college-aged daughter illustrates how kin relations can spark ethical reflection. Heather was a clinician and an instructor, and though this work was professionally satisfying, the dual positions meant that she was busy. She mixed her teaching responsibilities with twelve-hour shifts in a hospital. When I asked her how she decided to join her mission, she immediately said, "It was [my daughter]. She was like, 'You really should contribute to society, Mom' [laughs]. . . . It is really funny, but you know, I mean, I do have to say I think the younger generation is very tuned into the world and that they really feel [it is] really important to help out." She had thought about mission work before, but when she realized that most clinical placements in her field required a four- to five-month commitment, she dropped the idea until Sarah, her daughter, encouraged her to participate.

Heather began to consult with colleagues whom she thought might be able to help her find an appropriate placement that could accommodate her constraints. Due to the rhythm of her own professional life, she needed a mission that required a weeks-long commitment and that took place in the summer, when her teaching responsibilities were at a minimum. She needed a mission that could accommodate both her, as a clinical professional, and her daughter, a college student. She also wanted to find something geographically close, meaning in the Americas, as she did not want to waste time she could be volunteering traveling farther afield. Finally, she wanted something that would be safe, as she did not want to take Sarah anywhere risky. Eventually, her colleagues recommended the particular mission in which she and Sarah participated.

Heather's example highlights how kin ties influenced her decision to act. While Heather had imagined working internationally with an organization like Doctors Without Borders later in her career, her daughter's judgment of how much she was or was not contributing to society galvanized her own critical reflection of her current engagement and prompted Heather to seek out volunteering opportunities. While Heather initially felt good about her professional contributions and accomplishments, she soon agreed with Sarah that her ethical life was falling short. She wanted to find a way to give back now, in line with her values and aspirations. That Sarah was the one to point out her mother's shortcomings is also consequential. Heather not only valued

Sarah's commitments to doing the right thing but also admired who her daughter was becoming. It was Heather's responsibility to encourage her daughter to care about and take responsibility for others where possible. In this case, while the jornada gave Heather the option to practice professionally, the decision to participate immediately, rather than wait until a more convenient time, was made in relation to her ethical life. Heather's kin ties to Sarah changed the valence on her decision to volunteer or not volunteer.

Parent-child relationships commonly led parents to participate in STMMs in fulfillment of ethical commitments to their children. For example, parents talked about the importance of volunteering in missions as a way of teaching children about their own privilege and responsibility to society. Dana was a veteran of medical missions when she was recruited by her colleagues to go to Guatemala. What clinched the deal for her was that the mission would allow her daughter to join her. By the time I interviewed Dana, she had brought each of her kids with her on missions. She explained this to me by saying, "So I actually made an effort to take all my kids on various medical missions because I really— once I went, I saw that . . . it is an incredibly valuable experience for a young adult . . . who grew up in a very entitled, you know, comfortable setting to see how the rest of the world lives and how other people have it. I just think it's really eye-opening for them, and to me, it's just incredibly, incredibly valuable." While Dana had completed missions with each of her kids, Stephanie's kids were still too young to go. Nevertheless, Stephanie talked about why she wanted her children to accompany her on future missions, echoing Dana's reflection that going on missions could help her children understand their own privilege:

> I think that it would give them, one, a better perspective of what our world is actually like. We, as a family, . . . don't travel a lot. . . . In our lives, I feel like we grow up in this sort of—and the older we get, we develop blinders sometimes of, "This is what my world is." I want my kids to be able to see, when we go on vacations or when we do trips, life's not about Hawaii or Disney World. Although those things are so wonderful to go to, and I'm thankful that we get to go to those places, that there's other places in the world that just want to have clean water and food. Not getting so entitled in our own life of, "Well, I deserve this and that." To really

say, "This is my experience in my life. This is where I've gone to help other people. This is how they live." Life isn't just about the latest in fashion and clothing and vacations. That life is about more than that.

Dana's remarks begin to make evident the global dynamics that perhaps are more nascent in Heather's example. Again, drawing on Deomampo (2016), how kinship and volunteering connect to ethical life only begins to make sense when contextualized within volunteers' wider ideologies concerning global dynamics of privilege. North American volunteers were attuned to their own relative privilege as well as that of their children. Indeed, Stephanie's remarks most clearly articulate different visions of place that drive the global dynamics that underwrite volunteering. On the one hand, we have entitlement and vacation; on the other, we have places that need clean water and food. To live a good life, one must empathize with the experiences of others and, when possible, help those who are struggling. As Stephanie's quote shows and as Sarah made clear to her mom, giving back is essential to living an ethical life.

Stephanie's remarks illustrate how kin ties play a role in anchoring medical missions to volunteers' reflections on their ethical lives, or "how one should live and what kind of person one should be" (Keane, 2016:20). Not only are parents prompted by their children to live more ethically by volunteering (as their children define living ethically), but parents consider bringing their kids to volunteer as important early steps in fostering their children's ethical values. Children must see how people live in order to understand how they can effectively give back. Indeed, Dana, who had participated in numerous missions, was only prompted into action again because her daughter would be able to join her on this latest mission.

Finally, kin relations could also inspire a volunteer to act, even if kin stayed at home. Like Heather, Ana was introduced to the idea of international work with Doctors Without Borders, and, also like Heather, she said, "I'd taken a look and studied that outfit, and it was really long term. I knew that it wouldn't work." The time commitment was too extensive. Professionally, she could not leave her practice for months at a time; personally, she could not leave her family. Eventually she learned about her first STMM and realized that she might be able to manage it with the support of her family. Participating in a mission requires one's whole family to make sacrifices—she had to pay for her travel, she had to use her vacation time, her husband had to provide domestic labor and child care, and her children had to agree to manage without her. Ana described her husband's support by saying that he was "doing his own mission." She said, "If I'm gone and the kids are here, he'll manage that. . . . He's been incredibly supportive. I always say that it's almost like he's doing his own mission, staying at home while I go do my stuff." Indeed, Ana said about going on missions, "[It has] just been ingrained into our family life. They see how rewarding it is for me and the kind of things that I have done." She pointed to the fact that both of her children wanted to accompany her on these trips as soon as they were old enough. Indeed, when her son turned sixteen, he asked to attend the next mission with his mom.

For Ana, being part of a kin unit amplified the ethical dimensions of her mission work. While Ana was the one who was physically going on the missions, the mission work had become an intimate part of her family's ethical life and provided each of her family members an opportunity to live the kind to lives they wanted to live and be the kind of people they wanted to be. Her husband assumed all of the household responsibilities while Ana was gone not only out of necessity but willingly. This domestic work enabled his wife to provide her medical skills to people who they thought really needed them. In this way, it was "his own mission." Likewise, Ana's entire family accommodated the decrease in income and vacation time to allow Ana to care for others. Once again, this example highlights how kin relations can be integral to a volunteer's thinking about medical missions as part of ethical life. However, this example illustrates how, through kin relations, volunteering at a STMM can create a larger ethical footprint. Ana understands the ethical dimensions of her volunteering to include the support of her family, who stayed home.

Ana's story was echoed by a veteran STMM organizer who told me, "Some people go every year, and some people go every two or three years. Recidivism is real high because it's such a great experience. People want to share that with their family members and because it's a good experience for them. It also helps with the support 'cause nobody goes as an individual in this. I mean, it's a village kind of thing. For everybody who goes, there's a spouse at home taking care of the kids." While participating in STMMs may be a professional activity, kin relations can function as a type of ethical weather vane that prompts volunteers to consider particular professional activities as rich parts of their (and their families') ethical lives.

## Global Health as Profoundly Personal

How is participating in global health attractive enough to lure people into putting aside their full-time jobs and lives? The epigraph to this chapter leaves us with an account of global health activity that is both linear and skeletal, pairing a desire to give back with engagement. Popular essentialism suggests that global health work is a way of taking action to change the world for the better. This powerful essentialism is propagated by and remains consonant across the multiplicity of organizations that do global health work—be they private voluntary organizations, nongovernmental organizations, philanthropic endeavors, or even global initiatives like the UN's Sustainable Development Goals. Scholarship on global health that analyzes this trope of changing the world has fallen into a pattern of privileging the efficacy of global health: it takes for granted that action in the name of global health actually helps people it is intended to help, it dismisses the idea that this sort of action has created intended changes, or it suggest ways to enhance what is being done to better ensure desired changes. While questions of efficacy are important, they leave us focused on that original trope: whether or not global health action is changing the world as intended. I have intentionally tried to find a way to examine ethical dimensions of STMMs for volunteers that do not focus on efficacy. We must amplify the narrow focus set by popular essentialism to understand more deeply the contingencies that shape, enfranchise, and constrain contemporary global health practice.

The values and ends that drive volunteers toward global health work can be profoundly personal, and we miss this facet when we look only through a narrow lens. We miss how this kind of work connects to North American parents' tremendous efforts to cultivate gratitude in their children. We miss how it connects to parents modeling for their children how to address their own privilege. We miss how important unspoken (and perhaps unexamined) beliefs are to interpretations of action as unimpeachably good. It is these highly private and particular facets of life that make engaging in global health action important to volunteers as people, as well as make it the right thing for them to do.

Within the larger scope of this book, this chapter prepares us to reconsider connections between ethics, affect, and global health. Arguments of efficacy showing how global health action is tied to or reinforces systems of inequity may be useful in challenging organized, formal global health endeavors. However, these arguments are unlikely to extinguish the growing number of North American volunteers' interest in global health work. Such approaches underestimate how the connections between ethical lives and affect shape contemporary global health action, let alone how ethical lives and affect make DIY global health practically impervious to scholars' structural critiques. As we have seen, before the first patient is even seen, volunteers already had ideas about the ethical nature of global health work. In other words, what makes volunteers seek out particular modes of global health engagement, like STMMs, precedes and supersedes the global health domain; important elements, like kinship or race, that make global health action part of ethical life, come from outside the domain. Global health work can be profoundly personal. Moreover, the contribution of global health work to volunteers' ethical lives must be understood with reference to STMMs as a transnational practice (Deomampo, 2016). Indeed, it is not doing the work itself that creates value; the value comes when volunteers understand their work within a particular frame.

Furthermore, this chapter highlights the connections between ethical narratives that global-health-as-personal-work gives rise to and volunteers' feelings about that work—particularly feelings of achievement. The durability of these narratives further illuminates why I chose to consider Guatemala as a backdrop or idea of place. Guatemala appears to be fertile for ethical action precisely because it is a scene on a stage. For North Americans, volunteering at home can be more complicated—for example, because you can frequently understand the contextual environment in which a patient has failed to thrive (at least financially) and because you can identify patients' moral or dispositional failures, or because addressing an issue like access to health care through a stopgap measure like volunteering also may be less palatable in a jurisdiction where you can vote, particularly if you believe that health care is a human right. As we can see in this chapter, then, "flattening" Guatemala and not attending to its nuanced and complicated social and political past or present can contribute to volunteers' positive feelings about their actions.

Earlier chapters in this book explain how ethical action drives the work of STMM volunteers; the remaining chapters look more closely at the role of affect in volunteers' intimate reflections on their own actions. I argue not only that affect is important as a response to global health work but also that volunteers use their own affect to inform themselves of what is happening and what has happened during global health travel. Chapter 3 further explores the importance of affect in shaping contemporary global health by elucidating the relative strength of visceral feelings in defining the ethical value of global health action.

3

## Transformative Moments

### *"Body-Knowledge" and Ethical Action*

I must admit that it is very enticing to be here.
—my reflections about volunteering at a jornada taken from
my field notes

Antonia was a quiet K'iche' Maya woman from the outskirts of Nahualá whom I met while I volunteered at a short-term medical mission. She was petite, and it was not until you stood in front of her that you saw her problem; Antonia looked like she was beginning her third trimester of pregnancy. Unfortunately, she had looked this way for several years, yet no baby had been born. The surgeons at this weeklong jornada decided that Antonia had a mass that needed to be removed and scheduled her for surgery. She arrived with her father the day before her operation and settled into her bed. There was much speculation among mission volunteers, like me, and among the patients, who shared the recovery space with Antonia's family, regarding just what was wrong with her. Her front was enormous. The question everyone was asking was, "What is in there?"

Early in the morning, Antonia was taken into the pre-op room. Around lunchtime, I heard some patients saying that the surgeons had removed a mass from Antonia's abdomen. Though Antonia was not out yet, a volunteer had the mass in a plastic tub in the recovery room. Since I was going on break, I ran up to the recovery room to see what was going on. All the patients recovered in the same room, and it was stuffed with hospital beds. Next to each bed sat family members in plastic garden chairs. When I arrived, I saw that everyone who could walk had gathered around the volunteer, who was holding the plastic tub. I joined the crowd, trying to get a clearer view. When it was my turn in front, I saw that the tub contained a bloody yet discrete growth that I later learned was sixteen pounds of flesh. I would have expected to feel revulsion, but my reaction seemed aligned with those of my neighbors: the flesh was an object of amazement. As many patients in the recovery room were bound to their beds and could not see what we were looking at, the volunteer took the tub around the room, and the audible oohs and ahhs followed like a wave.[1] While we were watching, the Guatemalan woman beside me turned to me, awestruck, and remarked on the miracle it must have been to have that thing removed from you.

Later that night, after my shift had ended, I returned to the recovery room to talk to Antonia and found her accompanied by her father. As the other patients and families looked on, I asked Antonia if she could tell me about why she had decided to come to the jornada. She recounted to me that two weeks prior, an angel had come to her in her dreams and told her, "Don't worry, I'm going to see whom I can find to help you." On that day, Antonia started to pray for a cure. Then her sister told her about the medical mission and encouraged her to go. Antonia's father wept quietly during our conversation and then asked me if I had seen what the surgeons took out of his daughter. I told him I had. He had seen it too. He could not believe that his daughter had had to carry it around for so long and stressed to me the pain and bleeding that it had caused. He wept from relief that his daughter had found her cure. For Antonia's part, losing the sixteen-pound fibroid made her look almost like another person. Even sitting in bed on the same day of her surgery, she looked years younger.

Antonia's story reflects but one of my experiences at jornadas that has allowed me to think differently about ethical action in the domain of global health, as these experiences made me consider seriously the generative possibilities that emerge from embodied experience, leading to what I call "visceral ethics." Before volunteering, my thoughts on what constituted ethical action in Guatemala were influenced by my disciplinary background. My view of ethical action was tied to producing sustained well-being in Indigenous communities; this could be accomplished primarily by addressing ongoing issues of colonization, which produce the structures underlying injustices and thus hinder well-being and yield poor health outcomes (Jones et al., 2019; King, Smith, & Gracey, 2009). As discussed earlier, medical missions are not designed to be structural interventions and certainly do not systemically address colonization. As we have seen, medical missions arise from, if anything, a contemporary interpretation of global health that distances practitioners from the onus of considering colonialization in relation to their own actions. You can imagine my surprise, then, when I left missions *feeling* like the work I had done was integrally connected to my own ethical life. This chapter derives from my personal experience of volunteering in jornadas and traces how a small number of spectacular moments changed me and thereby reworked my understanding of how volunteers can constitute what they consider to be ethical action in global health.

The material in this chapter illustrates how my feelings supplanted my academic mode of understanding the ethical value of my personal action. I went from considering STMMs as silent on root causes of injustice at best and as contributing to ongoing injustice at worst to feeling awed and accomplished whenever I thought back to my work within a jornada. Please note that this is not a claim that my experience uncovered new evidence that rebutted or repositioned my academic knowledge; on the contrary, my academic position on ethical action remained intact. In other words, when I thought about working in a jornada, these gut feelings spoke far more strongly to me about my actions than what I knew to be problematic about STMMs from my academic research. In this chapter, I use my experience to build an argument that visceral ethics is a dominant mode to understand ethical action in DIY global health and thus an important force in the global health domain.

Why would centering myself and my feelings about my experiences lead me to consider a new mode of understanding action as ethical? Centering my own experiences created a different orientation toward how I learn about the world, enabling affect to become "epistemologically productive" (Stodulka, Selim, & Mattes, 2018). My past approaches to global health have been tied to typical modes of learning in the academy, including precisely articulated arguments, marshaled evidence, and scholarly debate. For me, centering my experiences and feelings effectively truncated the primary role of external input and debate in shaping my knowledge. Branwyn Poleykett (2016) points out that participant observation, like volunteering in a jornada, necessarily creates an opening for a researcher to acquire knowledge grounded in their own bodily experiences. This "body-knowledge" frequently generates different insights than knowledge generated through more traditionally academic means. To illustrate, I have read myriad columns in professional journals containing members' personal reflections of STMMs, many of which focus on moments of volunteers' transformations. I never recall being moved by any of them. Yet, when these moments occurred amid my own work in missions, I felt them quite profoundly, which has led me to understand them differently. Indeed, my body-knowledge about STMMs only became important to me because it conflicted with my academic knowledge.

The anthropologist Nora Jones's (2011) assessment of bioethics provides a different, yet complementary, explanation for why my own experiences might inspire novel understandings of ethical action. Jones's critique compares academic and experiential approaches to bioethics with reference to consideration of bodies. She points out that the typical academic approach to understanding ethics is to invent a hypothetical actor and then analyze their action in relation to certain principles. That actor, however, is a general, neutral somebody, not a real somebody with a particular experience.[2] Indeed, Jones argues that this academic tendency to depend on generic abstractions of people (and thus bodies) might limit our understandings of ethics. To illustrate, she tells us: "Many areas of concern for bioethicists, such as informed consent, advanced directives, or the mediation of a conflict over treatment options are considered as if the key players were disembodied rational actors" (Jones, 2011:73). Jones (2011:73) asks us, "Can . . . fleshing out . . . the players . . . make bioethics more ethical?"

After reading Jones's questions, I am convinced that the generic and reasoned are no more likely than the particular and idiosyncratic to determine our understandings of the ethical nature of our own actions. As demonstrated in chapter 2, our own places in the world and intimate relationships can influence how we perceive action taken as ethical. My experience working in STMMs highlights how body-knowledge can speak just as loudly as or even more loudly to us than our analytical minds do about what is right, wrong, just, and fair.

In what follows, I unpack what it was like for me to volunteer at a jornada. I begin by addressing the remarkable disjuncture between what I remember about my jornada work and what I recorded in my field notes. Doing so gives the reader a better sense of the work I did and also helps to highlight the stark disconnect that made me question what I was leaving out of my analysis when I first intended to write a book about STMMs. I then go on to chronicle some moments that were transformative. Despite their rarity, these moments are central to my gut feelings about jornadas and have become the anchor of the sense of purpose and ethical value that my gut reflexively associates with jornadas. I also explore dynamics that enable missions to produce such transformative moments and consider why these dynamics might be such an important part of the STMM environment and yet absent from other clinical environments where I have worked.

## The Highs and the Lows: What I Did and What I Remember about My Jornada Work

I participated in four different short-term medical missions in Sololá as a participant-observer. I was assigned an active work role, like everyone else at the mission. While I do not have any clinical skills, my linguistic fluency in Spanish and Kaqchikel Maya were assets because I could communicate in ways that many of the other volunteers could not. Thus, my roles were often connected to frontline communications with patients and their families. I could translate for clinicians, record patient histories, run the triage station, and so on. For me, mission work is characterized by never being alone. I was working and interacting with others continually while I fulfilled my roles.

Working at a jornada was frequently boring, always exhausting, and sometimes demoralizing. Indeed, every mission that I accompanied was, to some extent, a grueling experience. We would start early in the morning and end late in the evening. Since STMMs typically happen in spaces converted to accommodate them, we inevitably had to perform a daily setup and takedown. Unlike a hospital or a clinic where someone might be hired to do this sort of labor (e.g., sterilize important equipment, restock consumables), at a mission, the volunteers did this work.

Inevitably, we were busy trying to see everyone who wanted to be seen. Days when I interpreted back and forth between two people who could not communicate directly were exceptionally exhausting, as they required the most sustained focus. Other assignments were less mentally taxing and frequently included short bursts of activity that would be followed by long periods of waiting, as I would shuffle patients through a line, to triage, and then to a doctor.

The different days that I spent volunteering, and the cases that I saw, tend to bleed together in my memories. My field notes are full of cases that left little impression on me, and indeed I would have forgotten about them if I had not written them down. For example, one day I wrote about "the least satisfying case of the day," a woman who reported general pain all over the trunk of her body. She had visited a private doctor, who took some abdominal pictures on an ultrasound machine and told her that she needed surgery for her ovaries. Since she did not have enough money to pay the doctor for surgery, she decided to travel to the jornada to see if she could get her surgery there. The volunteers looked at her ultrasound pictures, which, instead of showing her ovaries, showed her kidneys and her gall bladder. They therefore did their own ultrasound and found nothing irregular in her ovaries or in her organs. They asked me to report to the patient that they did not know what was wrong with her.

At this point, the patient seemed flummoxed, so we sought out a Spanish-to-K'iche' translator (the patient's first language) to help with the consultation. The volunteers told me what to tell the K'iche' translator, who then talked to the patient to make sure she understood. After this multilingual game of Telephone, the K'iche' translator then asked, "Well, what should she do?"[3] The clinician said that the patient should try journaling about her pain. She should try to figure out if there were factors related to when she felt the pain (like activities or times of the day) and where exactly on her body she hurt. After I explained this, the translator asked, "And then what?" The clinician volunteer advised her to go back to a doctor to see if someone could help. In my field notes, I wrote that I found this encounter "a bit depressing." I felt disappointed because the patient had traveled from a town that was about five hours away by bus. Her investment of time and money to come to the jornada had resulted in naught. She already said that she did not have a lot of money, so the fact that we could not do anything for her depressed me. I also felt disappointed because I was skeptical that she had received helpful advice. First, I was not sure she could "journal." The idea of a journaling format, in which you record the date and reflective observations regarding descriptions of pain or body parts, seemed like a genre bounded by culture or access to institutional education that patients might not have enjoyed. Even if she could write, in everyday life in the town where I lived, paper, pens, and pencils were luxury items purchased on an as-needed basis, and there was certainly no guarantee that she had extra money to buy any of this. Second, being a poor, Indigenous woman in Guatemala was frequently not an easy life. It was possible that her nonspecific pain was more complicated than a particular malady that could be identified through journaling or cured through a follow-up clinical visit (for a related discussion of gender, social status, and pain, see Finkler, 1994). Finally, I wrote, given the ultrasounds that she brought with her to the jornada, I was suspicious of her doctor. Guatemala, like other countries where medical technologies have proliferated in the private sector (Gammeltoft & Nguyên, 2007), suffered from a problem of clinicians profiting from excessive testing and imaging. During my years of living in Guatemala, I had seen many unnecessary tests used to convince patients that they should spend additional monies on subsequent unneeded therapeutic interventions. Perhaps in this case the patient had misunderstood what her images were, or perhaps she lost an accompanying image of her ovaries. But perhaps her doctor was dishonest and was trying to take advantage of her pain to swindle her into paying him for an unneeded operation. Redirecting her back to the doctor could result in some sort of operation, making her poorer without addressing her underlying issues.[4]

My field notes are full of these sorts of cases that I marked as "unsatisfying" to me and that tended to consist of seeing patients with real complaints but whom we lacked the ability to help. For example, another day I prepared charts for many women who came with the same complaint—when they lifted up their arms, they had pain in their shoulders. When I asked how their pain started, each of the women answered that it was related to weaving. The women earned money by weaving cloth on their back looms at home. There was no ergonomics specialist who could visit their homes to help them adjust their work environment. No medical advice would alleviate their condition. Relief would only come for them if they stopped weaving or at least stopped weaving so much. But women needed to weave to earn money for their families. Reducing their workload—and therefore their income—was not a viable alternative.

Other notably unsatisfying yet common cases included women who came to the jornada due to excessive, smelly vaginal discharge or, sometimes, pelvic pain. They were usually diagnosed with sexually transmitted infections (STI) and given antibiotics to treat themselves and their partners. While diagnosing a woman with an STI was certainly valuable for her, it would have been preferable for us to speak to her partner too. If they both did not understand what had created the exposure and infection in the first place, they both might be reinfected. If he did not take the antibiotics, even if she was treated, she would be reinfected.

My *memories* of working in jornadas stand in stark contrast to what was recorded in much of my field notes. In my memories, the exceptional cases, not the grueling reality of my mission work, are what stand out. While I spent hours upon hours of exhausting work, much of it devoted to "unsatisfying cases" that I no longer remember, I would have recalled these exceptional, memorable cases even if I had not written about them. My memories of mundane experiences have fallen away; what remains are those that filled me with excitement, purpose, awe, and accomplishment. What I remember are the extraordinary and the miraculous cases, like that of Antonia.

While I was able to rush to the recovery room to view the mass that had been removed from Antonia, I missed many other cases that were almost as notable. For instance, one of the jornadas included a prosthetist, who fitted a patient who had lost his hand ten years before. Word had spread through the clinical space where I was working to make our way to the storage building to see the patient get his new hand. On my break, I followed the stream of patients and volunteers from many different stations, all rushing toward the storage building. The triage space, right next to the storage building, was notably empty as the patients and family members who were waiting to be seen had joined the migration. I merged into the crowd and waited for several minutes; but eventually my break was over, and I had to return to my post before the reveal. Nevertheless, I heard the story of what had happened after I left, retold both from the patients, who eventually returned to the clinic where I was working, and from other volunteers who had observed the event and retold the story later for those of us unable to witness it. Apparently, everyone had gathered around the patient in the storeroom and had watched as the prosthetist completed the final fitting. The prosthetist then handed the patient a pen and a piece of paper. Grabbing the pen with his new hand, the patient wrote his name for the first time in ten years. Everyone cheered. Then, underneath his name, he wrote the word *gracias* (thank you). The first time I heard that story, I remember my heart swelling with emotion and my eyes welling with tears. To me, in that moment, the way that the mission was able to change that man's life felt so profoundly good.

Another particularly awe-inspiring experience shared among missioners and between patients related to people who had (re)gained eyesight. Patients with cataracts would come in to have them removed. After surgery, their eyes would be taped over with gauze. When it was time to the remove the gauze, patients would return to the general clinic. Often, the gauze was removed in the waiting area, which was a far more generous space than the clinician's room. When I was able to see the gauze removed from one older man's eyes, I realized why so many people were talking about the experience. The older man instantly realized that his sight had returned and was reduced to tears of emotion. He was overjoyed to be able to see again and proceeded to grab and thank everyone around him. I did not know him personally, and I had not done anything to help him regain his sight; but I felt deeply connected to him, to his experiences, and to his joy. It was a blissful feeling. I also witnessed a three-year-old boy, who had never been able to see, have the gauze removed from his one operable eye while he sat in his mother's lap. The boy looked around and immediately burst into tears, grabbing his mother's blouse and burying his head in her chest while he wailed. The child was apparently surprised and overwhelmed; his parents were overjoyed. They hugged him, then tried to pull him out from hiding, all the while thanking the clinicians. Both of these instances inspired great emotion in patients, in the professionals who cared for them, and in the onlookers, like me, who had the fortune to witness such rare moments.[5]

These moments that I saw and remember carried unexpected and uncommon emotional weight. I felt included and involved in someone else's needed good fortune. These experiences felt uncomplicated; they made me feel good. They also connected me to the people with whom I was working, be they other volunteers, patients, or their family members. We were magnetized by the tiny miracles occurring around us, and we were drawn to share and witness as many as we could.

## Cultivating "An Experience" through the Spectacular

What is most remarkable about my memories of jornada work is that I do not have comparable memories of my prior research visiting clinics and working in the hospital in Sololá. Why can I detail so many of these high moments that I associate with working at jornadas but not those that I experienced in other health care settings? Certainly, in my prior research at the hospital, I witnessed events unparalleled in my life: doctors treating the damage wrought to flesh by the bite of a venomous brown recluse spider or a gunshot to the leg or the mayhem created when a public bus crashed into a car on the highway, flooding the tiny emergency room with bodies to be saved and the antechamber with keening relatives. Given that I was focused on obstetrics at that time, I also saw doctors save women from mortal birth-related complications. For example, I watched doctors prevent a deadly hemorrhage by removing the afterbirth still attached to a woman's womb. I also witnessed babies being born. Nonetheless, none of these experiences created the pure, simple euphoria of the memories that I associated with jornadas.

In examining humanitarianism in India, the anthropologist Erica Bornstein (2012:113) posits that, when volunteering "is uncoerced and selfless . . . it can lead to an 'experience.'" Drawing on Victor Turner, Bornstein renders an idea of experience that can be applied to my anecdotes: "Emerging from Turner's concept of 'social drama,' narratives of experience mark rites of passage. Thus, they refer to situations that are formative—not simply 'experience,' but 'an experience' that stands out. . . . Turner notes that such experiences 'erupt from or disrupt routinized, repetitive behavior' and 'begin with shocks of pain or pleasure.' He notes: 'The Greek peraō relates experience to "I pass through." In Greek and Latin, experience is linked with peril and experiment'" (Bornstein, 2012:113, quoting Turner, 1986:35). Seeing Antonia before and after her surgery and bearing witness to what was removed from her was, for me, "an experience." Bornstein tells us that the right moments can be "transformative" for volunteers.[6] Indeed, these experiences are characterized by strong affect, as I describe. In some cases, Bornstein finds, it is the affective dimension of having an experience that captures volunteers and keeps them in the humanitarian domain. As Bornstein notes, those who have "passed through" are frequently propelled to try to get others to volunteer.

I would suggest that at least part of the reason why jornadas created "an experience" for me is inextricably coupled with the fact that I was volunteering. Indeed, I have seen many tubs of afterbirth at the hospital (removing some of them prevented hemorrhaging and death), and none has ever created "an experience" the way that Antonia's flesh in a tub did. My research at the public hospital was immersive, but I did not feel implicated in care the way I did at the jornada. Certainly, in my earlier research, I was present during many care interactions, I was mistaken for a provider, and I helped translate and bridge the hospital systems for patients. Though I did not provide any medical care either at the hospital or at a jornada, I did have responsibilities for making care function at the jornada that I did not have at the hospital. I conclude that I witnessed Antonia's fibroid while positioned as a volunteer—it was this coupling that created "an experience" for me.

My lack of awe-inspiring experiences in regular clinics and hospitals has led me to reflect on how other dynamics of the jornadas contributed to my experiences. The overall ambiance of the hospital was wholly different for me. When I interviewed patients in the public hospital for this project, their focus was most typically on the *quality* of the care provided by doctors at the hospital. One of the interviewees who chose to have her hysterectomy in the public hospital characterized the hospital as "seguro," which in this context translated to indicate that it was both "safe" and "secure." Indeed, though chronically underfunded, care at the public hospital in Guatemala is guaranteed: the right of all citizens to health is enshrined into the constitution, so public care is always there and, theoretically, always free.[7]

Yet, as the anthropologist Elysée Nouvet (2016) and Stephanie Roche et al. (2018) have documented in both Nicaragua and Guatemala, patients at STMMs are full of gratitude. There were explicit expressions of thankfulness and indebtedness and comments on the goodness of the volunteers. Some convalescing patients explained that, while they were poor and therefore could not pay money for private care, God would pay their debt. Others were more direct in offering their own benediction ("Que Dios le bendiga," or "May God bless you"). Even when Antonia recounted her own experience, it was angels who sent the surgeons to Guatemala to help her. In short, patients in jornadas both drew attention to and remarked on their caregivers' goodness or deservingness.[8]

For me, when working at a jornada, a sense of being good or deserving was associated with being a volunteer—and this emanated both from patients and from other volunteers.

From where does this expression of gratitude come, and why was it prevalent at jornadas? The anthropologist Jessaca Leinaweaver (2013) reminds us that expressions of gratitude or ingratitude often map back onto larger social structures, though, as Nouvet (2016) points out, it can do so without critiquing inequities. In the hospital, patients receive care as part of their rights; outside of the public system, patients always have to offer something for their care. Most of the time, the offering comes in the form of a fee that must be paid to the provider. Remember Carmen, whom we met earlier, who sat down and immediately asked how much she would be charged to be seen at the jornada? Indeed, this was not an infrequent question from people who were waiting for or receiving care at the jornada.

Traditionally anthropological analyses of the giving of gifts, like free care at a jornada, have emphasized how gift giving engenders exchange, meaning that the recipient of a gift is now indebted to the giver of the gift (Mauss, 1990).[9] When we read the provision of care at a jornada as an exchange, it seems to make sense that patients' blessings might be not only their sincere expressions of gratitude but also attempts to reciprocate. They have been given a gift of care, and they offer blessings and compliments on the goodness of the givers in exchange.

For me, being part of an environment in Sololá with such a palpable expression of gratitude was surprising, especially because before I started working at jornadas, both Indigenous and non-Indigenous Guatemalans often expressed skepticism of the idea that jornadas were about helping patients per se. In attempts to shed doubt on the moral integrity of STMMs, Guatemalan interviewees frequently proposed that jornadas actually profit volunteers and suggested that the stories about jornadas' benevolence were used to provide moral cover for more selfish endeavors.[10] As noted earlier, clinicians and organizers often critiqued evangelical missions as self-serving. Similarly, Guatemalan health practitioners who saw the fallout of STMM care gone awry often asserted that volunteers were there to practice medical techniques that they were not allowed or able to practice at home. According to these local critics, jornada volunteers then took their improved clinical skills back to North America, where they could translate them into better care for their own patients, relinquishing any responsibility for the patients whom they practiced on in Guatemala.[11] Guatemalan interviewees who were broadly aware of the economy associated with North American NGO giving were on the lookout for how STMMs might be money-making businesses disguised as philanthropies. One interviewee told me to investigate the logistics that arose to support volunteering. Every jornada volunteer needed a room, board, transport, translation services, and so on. They were certain that organizers who sponsored jornadas were middlemen, profiting from the difference between the real costs of these amenities and the slightly inflated prices that they charged the volunteers. Moreover, when I casually described my research to Guatemalans I met during the course of my everyday life, they immediately focused on financial issues, quizzing me about whether volunteers were getting paid, where the money to send them was coming from, and why, if they were not getting paid, they would come to Guatemala. In short, many Guatemalans expressed skepticism of the narrative that jornadas were simply characterized by generous volunteers donating time, money, and expertise to help people they did not know.

Nevertheless, I found that, when on a jornada, any skepticism—my own and that of other volunteers—was muted and replaced by a sense of idealism. It was very important to most volunteers that, within the context of the jornada, care be given for free.[12] Indeed, there was an all-hands-on-deck spirit at the jornada that was dissimilar to the public hospital or other clinic environments I was familiar with in Guatemala, where health care workers struggled constantly with excessive demands on their time and faced a strict hierarchy. In contrast, at the jornada, everyone pitched in to work together. When trying to characterize how special this aspect of the jornada environment felt, one volunteer interviewee related an example of how all volunteers, regardless of status, made sure that the speculums were sanitized daily.[13] I also recall observing one seasoned volunteer clinician pull aside another new volunteer clinician to reorient them. The new volunteer was trying to recruit an assistant to clean the workspace between patients and to bring patients to them. The seasoned volunteer explained that everyone had to carry their own weight, which meant doing things that you were not normally responsible for in your own practice. The new volunteer quickly pivoted and adjusted their expectations. With everyone contributing, every volunteer felt just as responsible and indispensable as every other volunteer—that certainly echoes how I felt about my volunteer work.

Another common and inescapable difference between the hospital and the jornada was that the jornada was full of people like me: foreigners. In Guatemala, as elsewhere, medical encounters frequently happen between two strangers. But the strangers, often varied across class and race lines, are typically both Guatemalan. Yet, in the jornada, not only was care being given by strangers, but the strangers were relatively high-status foreigners, from high-income countries, and frequently White. As a White North American woman, I fit in at the jornada in a way that I did not when conducting participant observation at the hospital; and this was obvious to both patients and other volunteers.

Mike's story highlights how foreignness plays a role in coupling volunteering and "an experience." Mike accompanied a jornada and worked on a stove project, where he installed a new, wood-efficient, smoke-minimizing stove in a Mayan family's home. He began his tale by highlighting that he was not someone who easily feels "kinship" and "connection" with others; indeed, he pointed out that this was something that he had struggled with in the past. While he was installing the stove, creosote from the chimney fell onto his face, so that when he took off his glasses, he looked like a raccoon. He said that once he removed his glasses, the old woman and the children in whose home he was working laughed and laughed, and then they gave him some towels to wipe his face. When they did, they noticed how much hair he had on his arms and they started to pull it. He said, "Hey! I am connected to that hair!" though they could not understand him. Because Mike was hairier than your average Guatemalan and his audience was so impressed with his arm hair, he decided to show them his chest hair, which made them all laugh even more. The interaction paved the way for what came next. After the stove was installed, they took a picture, and when they did, Mike felt the small arm of one of the little girls winding around him. Savoring that little arm hugging him, Mike felt a unique connection to that little girl. That he could feel that connection was incredibly important for him. As he put it, it was not something that normally "happened" for him. In the parlance of North American volunteering, this was "an experience."

Mike's story helps show how volunteers' identities as North Americans contribute to the environment of a jornada and, therefore, help create "an experience." In Guatemala, foreigners function outside of typical social dynamics. In this case, a Guatemalan can pull a foreigner's unfamiliar body hair, but it is difficult to imagine that this would have happened if the stove installer had been an unusually hairy Guatemalan man. Here, not only could a Guatemalan pull a foreigner's arm hair, but she could do so with the confidence that it would not lead to anger or a violent reprisal. And indeed, Mike responded by hamming it up and showing them his chest. It is important to pay attention to the family's expectations here—certainly, their interaction with Mike was free of the judgments that they expected of their neighbors or other Guatemalans. Moreover, they approached the interaction anticipating not just random unexpectedness but something positive.

Volunteers' identities as North Americans are important to the ambiance created at a jornada. In Guatemala, North Americans are special types of strangers. My fellow North Americans and I have access to wealth. Guatemalans learn this through consuming mass media, observing the myriad tourists who appear to pay easily for expensive vacations, and noticing the dynamics of jornada and volunteer work more generally: North Americans travel to Guatemala not only to work for free but to give stuff away. North American volunteers and their activities are therefore bathed in a light of potential abundance, and jornadas are a mode through which Guatemalans get the chance to participate in or access some of that abundance. As Leinaweaver (2013) has argued, expressions of gratitude often accompany situations in which the perception is that the relatively poor and rich are brought together. In jornada interactions, gratitude abounds.

When I consider the differences in my experiences between watching lifesaving procedures in the hospital and surgeries in the jornada, the fact that I was a volunteer receiving gratitude in the latter, but not the former, is hugely significant. That light of potential abundance that shined on me at the jornada dimmed when I was at the public hospital. The jornada offered me a group of peers, patients, and families who saw my actions as good; this was also missing during my time at the hospital. Indeed, if the cases that I saw at the jornadas had been cases I witnessed at the hospital, where it was the staff's job to attend to them, I doubt that they would have constituted "an experience." How people saw me influenced how I felt about the moment. Getting to witness those cases, as a volunteer, in conditions prompted by a jornada, was what produced their affective weight for me.

## Body-Knowledge and Ethical Action

How does body-knowledge function as a finding from my research? It highlights the potential for affect to profoundly influence a volunteer's understanding of their own ethical action. In my case, the body-knowledge I derived from "an experience" contributed greatly to my gut feeling that volunteering for an STMM was good. Despite the fact that "experiences" I had might have constituted only one brief moment in a sea of intense work, they have proved obdurate. My gut feeling of what I did as good endures, years later. Furthermore, my gut feeling still defies my efforts to align it with my academic understanding of ethical action and how STMMs might fall short.

As suggested earlier, DIY global health work is generally considered work that fits well into volunteers' ethical lives. Volunteers' positive judgments of global health work are assumed to derive from having contributed to or created something positive in the world. But that is not how visceral ethics works. There was no causal relationship for me—my feelings of having taken action important to my ethical life did not derive from belief or systematic evidence that STMM work was good or important. My affective and academic experiences remain disparate. I find myself holding two different interpretations (one in my mind, one in my gut), both of which seem "true" to me.

Again, the material in this chapter reinforces the point that critical scholars, such as anthropologists, must broaden our scope if we wish to expand our understandings of global health. That affect does not reside in relation to analytical understandings typical to academia makes our current hyperfocus on structures in global health problematic. Focusing so heavily on global health as an equity-producing action (or not) privileges typical academic modes of knowing over affect as the mode through which we should understand global health. This approach eclipses important underlying affective forces that are equally consequential in shaping global health action as reasoned planning and judgment, if not more so. Chapter 4 further reveals the influence of visceral ethics on volunteers' intimate relation to their own actions.

4

# Lack of Context

*Why We Rely on Visceral Ethics in DIY Global Health Work*

As volunteers spoke with me about their global health work, several mentioned award-winning, nonfiction writer Tracy Kidder's (2003) biography of the physician-anthropologist Paul Farmer, *Mountains beyond Mountains: The Quest of Dr. Paul Farmer, a Man Who Would Cure the World.*[1] Kidder's exploration of Farmer's life and work does an excellent job of inspiring us to see "how one person can make a difference in solving global health problems," as so poignantly summarized on the back jacket of my dog-eared copy.[2] Notable are the descriptions of Farmer's dedication to caring for strangers across the world as if they were his own family.

Years before participants talked to me about Farmer, the medical anthropologist David Citrin (2011) had already written about *Mountains beyond Mountains* and its role in recruiting clinicians to pursue global health work. He noted that Farmer "has become an animating force that (intentionally or otherwise) peddles the experience of a particular kind of global health narrative. . . . His aura now serves as a catalyst for the flow of short-term medical volunteers in the form of clinicians and students who are in search of doing good; who head out in search of curing their own worlds" (Citrin, 2011:27). Demonstrating this point in another way, when one interviewee was asked to describe what motivated him to volunteer for a STMM, he glibly told Citrin (2011:119), "Paul Farmer made me do it." Farmer works as "an animating force" for STMM volunteers because, as noted earlier, volunteering for an STMM is typically part of a volunteer's ethical life. Indeed, volunteers envision working at an STMMs as an action reflective of their values—they are, in Citrin's words, "in search of doing good."

In this chapter, I dig down deeper into how we can come to feel that our everyday actions are good work. My own prodding of Luz to get surgery at the jornada to fix her prolapse illustrates the potential gap between everyday actions that I myself am propelled to take because they are reflective of the kind of person I want to be and actually doing good. I ripped off that little piece of paper about the jornada from the telephone pole and took it to Luz because I wanted to be trustworthy. I told her that I was going to keep my eyes open for help after she asked me to. Yet upon reflection, I do not think that following through with my action increased my trustworthiness. On the contrary, it might have compromised it. Luz learned that if I make a commitment, I might meet the letter of the agreement but not the spirit. I did follow through on my promise to look for opportunities for her, but it is hard to argue that, by taking her to a jornada, I helped her. Indeed, perhaps the best judgment of whether my action was helpful—or "good"—comes from Luz herself. After the jornada experience, Luz never returned to me for help. Indeed, the last time I saw Luz was at a market a few years ago; though we both smiled and said, "Hi," we did not stop to chat. In short, we might take actions because we see them as integrally related to the type of person that we want to be, but that does not mean that just by taking action, we actually become that person.

This distinction between an intent to live a good life and a focus on whether the decisions that I make produce the good I seek to create on an everyday level was marked in my data. While volunteers with whom I worked overwhelmingly expressed being driven by an intent to do good (in other words, a clear component of ethical lives), many had more fine-grained concerns with fraught, unneeded, or ultimately damaging action taken under the guise of helping. Phillipe's experience in his first jornada to Guatemala, discussed earlier, is a good example—while he was clear in his intent to help through medical missions, he felt that his participation in a jornada in which he only rendered medical attention to patients who promised to convert to a certain religion was morally suspect.[3]

The anthropologist Cheryl Mattingly (2014) reminds us what Phillipe knows: trying to live a virtuous life is difficult and potentially perilous. As no one's ability to lead a virtuous life is foretold, Mattingly (2014:127) demands that we attend to how moral action is necessarily fraught with "frailty and uncertainty." She insists that we remain aware of the potential for individuals to face "moral tragedy, situations in which good people come to act in ways that they would otherwise reject, to do bad

things, because of circumstances they did not initiate and whose consequences they did not or could not foresee" (Mattingly, 2014:128). As both
Phillipe and I have learned, taking action intended to do good makes
you "morally vulnerable" because that action might unintentionally lead
to harm as easily as to good. The intention to do good therefore places
volunteers in moral peril—that is, puts them at a grave risk for doing
harm instead of good.

Mattingly cites Aristotle to bring forward the importance of context
to judgments of whether our action is good. Aristotle asserted that,
rather than being born into a good life, an individual cultivates the virtue necessary for a good life through practice. Ultimately the judgment
of our lives as virtuous (or not) stems from the sum of judgments of our
actions. Mattingly (2014:127) points out that Aristotle calls for "situated
*judgment* rather than an application of general rules to a particular case"
(emphasis in original). The ability to judge an action by general rules
allows us to determine if an action is righteous or not in all cases. For
example, a rule might be that global health action is necessarily good
action. Accordingly, in these conditions, if I judge that the action I took
was in fact in the domain of global health, I could necessarily judge it
as good. Situated judgments, by contrast, require a completely different
empirical inquiry to determine the moral valence of an action. Unlike
general rules, where actions are classed together, situated judgments require that every action be judged as a particular case. This is because the
same action taken by the same person could lead to harm in one case
and lead to good in another. The difference between the two can only be
determined in context.[4]

And here we arrive at the theme of this chapter: the importance of
context in judging the ethical nature of one's own action. The first half
of the chapter tracks the experiences of a global health veteran, Teresa,
a clinician whose long-term engagement in Sololá predates my own. Teresa self-admittedly was inspired by a desire to help people in Sololá,
and, like Paul Farmer, this was arguably a deep part of her ethics. Her
familiarity with context helps highlight how the ethical value of action
is context dependent. As Mattingly warns us, Teresa's experience demonstrates that global health action always bears a threat of harm, even
when an actor is well informed about context. I then examine several
instances in which interviewees (including Teresa) warned of harm with

regard to jornada volunteers' actions. Ultimately, I use a global health veteran's knowledge of Sololá and medicine to bring into relief how relying on ideas of place can create morally perilous situations for the short-term volunteers who come—situations of which they frequently might not even be aware until after the fact, if ever at all.[5]

The work that this chapter does for my overall argument is manifold. The examples brought forward help specify what I mean by context as well as how it might be instrumental to differentiating if one's action creates harm or good. This chapter also lays the first seeds of understanding how DIY global health places volunteers in moral peril as more than just an abstract concern. As North Americans are inundated with the idea that DIY global health is good, for some, the harm it can produce may be difficult to conceptualize. Yet, in this chapter, we can see how action taken at an STMM has the real potential of contributing to patients' deaths (rather than recovery or flourishing). I return to the importance of acknowledging the harm that can come from DIY global health in the book's conclusion. Finally, this chapter also contributes an important building block to my argument that visceral ethics is a central form of meaning-making for DIY global health volunteers, like those who attend STMMS. It draws into question short-term volunteers' ability to actually judge the impacts of their actions. As Mattingly points out, without understanding context, volunteers' judgments of their own actions cannot be *situated*. Without the ability to sufficiently understand context to situate judgments about moral action, STMM volunteers rely on visceral ethics to acquire certainty that the work that they did at a jornada constitutes good moral action.

## What to Do Next? Building a Good Life on Good Action

Teresa spent her entire medical career bouncing back and forth between her paid appointment as a trauma surgeon in a hospital in Texas and her volunteer medical work in Sololá. She was the first person to tell me to research medical missions when we met in 2003, while I was researching the Safe Motherhood Initiative. As someone who had worked for many years in the public hospital in Sololá, she was upset by the failed medical care provided by jornada volunteers that she had seen on several occasions. Yet over a decade later, when I contacted her about this project, I was surprised to learn that she had started working with jornadas during the past several years. Despite her status as a jornada volunteer, there was nothing "short term" about Teresa's engagement, and her role in this book is not to represent a typical DIY volunteer. Rather, Teresa's long-term engagement helps us see consequences of moral action that are often missing from accounts of actions taken at STMMs, as well the importance of context in determining whether action was helpful or harmful.

Teresa was drawn to Guatemala by her husband, Finn, a European who first traveled to the country as a young surgeon in the 1970s. His European medical license did not allow him to practice legally in Guatemala. He remedied this by completing an additional three-month residency in the main public hospital in Guatemala City, which secured his official status as a surgeon in the country. Early in his career, Finn took frequent vacations from his paying job in the United States, where he also had a medical license, to return to Guatemala to practice medicine. When Finn started working in Sololá in the 1970s, Guatemala was in the throes of civil war, and the Sololá public hospital was located in the war-torn western highlands. The hospital did not have medical specialists, so no staff member was equipped to handle many of surgical cases. But Finn was.

While working in Texas, Finn met Teresa, a Mexican national who had completed her surgical training in the United States. They married. In the early 1980s, Teresa began to accompany Finn to Sololá. The hospital director, with whom they built a positive relationship, trusted Teresa and Finn to attend surgical cases that he would normally refer to a hospital in the capital city. They each also gave continuing education courses to general doctors on hospital staff—Teresa in trauma care and Finn in internal medicine.

Up to this point, Teresa's narrative was essentially straightforward, but things started to change when the civil war in Guatemala came to an end in the mid-1990s. The Ministry of Health made it a priority to expand access to care and began to place Guatemalan specialists as interns in hospitals like the one in Sololá. By this time, however, the hospital was, as Teresa put it, "in total neglect." As patients' access to specialist care from her Guatemalan colleagues increased, she felt she could better contribute if she shifted some of her own attention to improving the decaying infrastructure in which she and her colleagues had to work.

While this would have been a simple undertaking in a private hospital, using private money on infrastructure in a public hospital is complicated in Guatemala. Article 94 of the Guatemalan constitution (Guatemala, 1985) establishes that it is the state's responsibility to work through its own institutions to "procurar [a todo los habitantes] el más completo bienestar físico, mental y social" (to promote the best physical, mental, and social well-being for all of its inhabitants). Arguably, allowing private investment to support public hospitals invites the state to abrogate its own responsibilities. Individuals or organizations must meet many thresholds to work though the state system, which forces them to spend a significant amount of time building relationships and navigating bureaucracies. Teresa had to form a Guatemalan NGO, Patronato del Hospital (Hospital Trust), the only legal function of which was to help the hospital. Teresa could donate money to the Patronato, which could then legally donate that money to the hospital. Once receiving the funds, the hospital acquired full legal dominion over their allocation. In other words, if the hospital decided to spend all of the donated money on toilet paper, this was perfectly legal, and neither the Patronato nor Teresa could object.

Given Teresa's history and relationships with the hospital director and staff, she trusted that they could work together to direct changes. For her first project, she set about to improve the emergency room. As Teresa describes it, at that time, "it was all just a big room, wide open and filthy," and it lacked equipment. Teresa worked on a "redesign" that could create private treatment areas and have necessary equipment organized and available. Once she had finished her plans, she presented it to the staff, which approved them. The director then took those plans to Guatemala City, where he presented them to Ministry of Health officials. They sent engineers and other representatives to the hospital to evaluate the proposed redesign and eventually approved the project. Teresa donated to the Patronato, the Patronato transferred the money to the hospital, and the hospital directorate paid for the project to be undertaken.

When I first met Teresa, she and Finn were checking up on the redesign. It was January 2003, and it was my first week of fieldwork in the public hospital, which was an important field site for my research. I was sitting beside the entrance to the emergency department, and I heard a new, commanding voice entering from the exit door. Soon, a man and woman wearing long, white doctors' coats appeared. I remember my first impressions: he was quite tall; she had presence. They handled themselves differently from everyone else. Teresa walked straight over to the shower curtain that was suspended from the ceiling to create a border between the patient in Bay 1 and the rest of the room. She examined the curtain, pulling it back and forth, looking at the front and back, and calling out her observations to Finn. I did not know who these people were; I did not know why she was so interested in the shower curtain. But the shower curtain should have taught me the first thing that I needed to learn about Teresa: she was a problem solver. In fact, I later learned that she had worked in that emergency department enough to decide that the lack of privacy was hindering care and that hanging shower curtains would be a simple and inexpensive solution. So she made it happen.

Teresa estimates that she had about four good years working with the Patronato. She took on projects that could improve conditions for patient care, including purchasing equipment (like an ultrasound machine) and redesigning spaces to make them more functional (like a small overflow operating room and a neonatology unit). When I interviewed her for this project, she did not focus on any of those aspects of her work with the Patronato and the hospital. Instead, she focused on actions she had undertaken without sufficiently understanding the wider context: her attempt to establish an intermediate care unit.

At that time, the public hospital in Sololá was divided into different wards. Depending on the time of day or the ward, one or two nurses could be responsible for tens of patients. Because of the nursing shortage, nurses were not expected to accompany or check on patients regularly. For many patients, this level of care was sufficient, but for others, such as, for example, those who had just come out of surgery, this was problematic. Teresa explained to me that outcomes for these patients could be significantly improved through more continuous care. She envisioned an intermediate care unit where the patients who needed more intensive treatment and monitoring could be placed together and receive more consistent care. She again worked with the hospital directorate to redesign a space, and then through the Patronato, she donated funding to equip that space for its new purpose.

Teresa soon learned that establishing a functional intermediate care unit was not merely a problem of infrastructure. Certainly, the hospital needed a redesigned space and new equipment. However, a successful intermediate care unit depended on nurses providing a different level of care to patients. Teresa viewed this as a technical problem. Her solution was to retrain the nurses and show them how to best use the space to care for patients.

The nurses, however, were concerned that their work conditions were deteriorating. They were being asked to provide more intensive, specialized care than they had been hired for. They saw this retraining for further professional specialization and assignment to the intermediate care unit as additional work. They wanted a pay increase to recognize this. Teresa agitated for two years to resolve these differences between the directorate and the nurses to help bring the intermediate care ward online. During that time, two of the expensive, new beds in the ward disappeared (Teresa suspected that they were stolen and sold). From Teresa's perspective, the intermediate care unit "caused a big to-do because all the nurses said, 'Well, we're not going to take care of intermediate care if they're not going to pay us, and we're not qualified. We don't know how to do it.'" Though we spoke about this more than a decade after it happened, Teresa was still frustrated. Her disgruntled translation of the nurses' resistance was, "It's better that the patients die than that we learn anything." When the directorate and the nurses finally reached an agreement and the ward became operational, she had had enough: "It had been about twenty-two or so years that I had been working there. Then, I said, 'You know what? This is for the birds.'" So she quit the Sololá hospital and closed down the Patronato.

Teresa's recounting of her experience with the Patronato highlights her moral vulnerability—in acting to create what she judged to be positive change, she potentially encouraged the opposite. While her retelling of this story does not delve deeply into the politics of the hospital, it raises concerns about how her action might have perturbed fragile relations. The resistance met from the nurses exposed factionalism between the administration, which approved and encouraged Teresa's plans, and the nurses, who were responsible for implementing them. Her efforts to create intermediate care also might have ended up fomenting corruption—the suspicious disappearance of the new beds. Both factionalism and corruption in turn could make it more difficult for patients at the hospital to get quality care. For example, if nurses feel undermined instead of supported by the administration, they may be less willing to invest in excellent care for patients. Furthermore, like many parts of the public sector in Guatemala, the hospital struggled with rumors of corruption. Increased corruption could make professionals wary of becoming involved in the hospital and make patients less trusting of their care providers. In Teresa's judgment of the nurses' action, she obliquely refers to the worst of tragedies—that, ultimately, her attempt to implement positive change might have resulted in negative change: patients receiving even worse care than they would have had she done nothing.

Though Teresa continued to fight until the intermediate care unit was functioning, the fact that she quit immediately afterward speaks to the uncertainty of this situation. She evidently did not think that getting this one unit up and running created an environment that assured the positive change that she envisioned. On the contrary, she decided that having to undertake such a struggle was "for the birds" and turned her attention toward a safer bet. In reflecting on this experience, Teresa recounted, "I think that in the . . . enthusiasm of the beginnings, we got overenthusiastic and overdid it a little bit."

While working in the hospital, Teresa had been privy to many cases resulting from missions gone awry. Nevertheless, as surgical missions became more routine in Sololá over the ensuing decade, Finn and Teresa built relationships with jornadas, too. They worked with many missions, sometimes on a one-off basis and other times participating throughout. Some missions asked them to join as surgeons or fill in for last-minute vacancies. Ultimately, Teresa and Finn found their niche in providing follow-up care once the missioners had left Sololá. She said, "I worked with a bunch of groups, lately, with just one or two. We have volunteered to do follow-ups, which is probably the best [thing] we have been able to do. The follow-ups are for [STMMs] that come and stay ten days, and then, they do the surgery and leave the patients pretty much floating in the wind. We will stay a week or two or three even and make sure that [everything is okay]." Finn and Teresa were uniquely placed to provide follow-up care, given their medical skills, their deep familiarity with available health care resources in Sololá and Guatemala in general, their connections with a variety of clinics and practitioners, their willingness to be in Guatemala for long periods of time, and their linguistic skills (fluency in medical English and Spanish). After years of collaboration, Teresa felt overall that "there is a lot of good that comes from these jornadas that [North Americans] do."

While Teresa's original trepidation regarding jornadas had subsided, she nonetheless commented on how jornada surgical work was fraught with potential peril. The first thing that she pointed out was the personnel organization characteristic of many STMMs: "I think the big thing [is] just the way people pass—the patients pass through—how do you say this—too many hands. One translates. The other examines. They're trying to include too many people. If it's a surgery jornada, by God, have surgeons and anesthesiologists and maybe one internist for consultations, but don't cut down on the work [of the surgeon], because you lose. You lose knowledge of the patient." My experiences working in jornadas affirms Teresa's accounts. Jornadas are frequently organized to identify as many patients as possible who need surgery. Benches full of patients wait to have their vitals recorded. Multiple people are screening patients for one type of surgery. Though I did not work in the operating room, I can imagine that a similar model might govern what happens there. For example, a nurse might be responsible for taking patients' vitals before the surgery, or another doctor may have performed a physical, rather than the scenario that Teresa recommends, in which the surgeon and the anesthesiologist are in the room together taking blood pressure and evaluating the patient prior to surgery. Teresa was worried that this practice of "trying to include too many people" would lead the surgeon to "lose knowledge of the patient."[6] She deemed this knowledge loss as risky for both the surgeon and the patient: "I will examine my surgical patients from stem to stern . . . by myself, and then, I'm comfortable operating on them, especially since I know I don't have any backup up there. It's me. . . . I'd say, 'Oh, my God. I really don't want to get into any trouble here because [there's] nobody [else]—that's it. It's Finn and [me].' That taught me to be absolutely super responsible. Maybe that is my big—one big hurdle from all the years that I've been up there [i.e., Sololá], the act of who makes sure of your patient. . . . You be sure."

Teresa's reflection that she could not rely on backup medical staff to perform preoperative examinations highlights a structural conundrum that creates moral vulnerability for individuals engaged in STMMs. DIY global health represents an opportunity for volunteers to take their professional expertise to a context that is decidedly different from what they are used to in multiple ways. These volunteers must therefore judge the right balance between relinquishing and retaining expertise in a new environment. For example, Teresa points out in her quote that many volunteers judge that it is appropriate to relinquish direct communication with the patient yet retain the ability to surgically remove an ovarian cyst. Others judge this situation appropriate when the full corporal examination of the patient has been at least partially outsourced. But for Teresa, this is morally culpable. As she says, "You be sure." To be clear, Teresa is asserting that you should not depend on others to evaluate or care for your patient in ways that you normally would in your home practice. Teresa's remarks also point to the moral peril associated with practicing biomedical interventions across different geographies. She talks about "all of the years that I have been up there," referring to her long history of practicing medicine in Guatemala.[7] There are elements of care that existed in her work in Texas that were not available in Guatemala. She points to being intimately familiar with the context of the wider medical setting as imperative for being able to do good work for her patients—you have to know what help is available and what help is not. Indeed, the moral imperative of being sure for yourself did not only guide her STMM practice. For much of her career in Guatemala, Teresa worked to achieve good outcomes for her patients by managing as much of the process as she possibly could. If she could not do a surgery successfully by herself, she would not do it.

Like Teresa, Guatemalan health professionals in Sololá told me stories confirming that this distributed form of care (what Teresa characterized as "not being sure") puts volunteers in moral peril. They continually circled back to two different instances of botched mission surgeries to make the point that slotting into the doctor role in a different country was not sufficient to ensure good patient care and, thereby, good and ethical action. To put this in a temporal context, each of these interviewees referred to incidents that occurred before Teresa encouraged me to research jornadas. These incidents are infamous enough that, though they happened years ago, Guatemalan interviewees still used them as touchpoints to show why jornadas were problematic.

One instance relates to a time when a jornada commandeered the Sololá public hospital operating rooms to do its surgeries.[8] Despite its physical location in the hospital space, no local doctors participated in jornada surgeries, patients operated on were not listed on the regular hospital rosters, and the jornada team brought its own nurses for case management. After surgery, patients recovered in the regular hospital wards (e.g., men's ward or women's ward). While the jornada staff attended to the patients throughout the afternoon, at the end of a long day, the team left.[9] The missioners assumed that their patients would be monitored by the regular on-duty night-shift hospital nurses.

Considering Teresa's difficulties starting an intermediate care unit at this hospital with limited staff, what happened next should come as no surprise. When the team returned in the morning to check on how everyone was recovering, they found that the jornada patients had not been attended by local nurses during the night. One patient had bled to death.

This example illustrates the important role of context in situated judgments as well as volunteers' reliance on visceral ethics to establish whether their own moral action is virtuous or perilous. In this case, the specific surgery was successful; nevertheless, the patient died. Teresa said, "You be sure," but we see how volunteers' judgments of being "sure" that they were taking care of their patient were insufficient, as these judgments ended the patient's life rather than bettered it. The volunteers were "sure" that there were hospital staff; their judgments of due diligence did not extend to ensuring that available staff would care for their surgical patients, let alone confirm how frequently or adequately they would attend to them. While this truncated understanding of being "sure" might have been adequate in Canada or the United States, the example highlights how working in STMMs is far more morally perilous for volunteers than practicing at home is. Not only, as Teresa says, is there no "backup there," but the facets of practicing in unknown contexts, such as where wards are short staffed or where patients have had no access to routine care, introduces a dimension of moral vulnerability, as STMM volunteers do not know what they do not know.

A second example highlights how difficult situational judgments become when volunteers find themselves in contexts different from where they normally work. As recounted in the prologue, my Guatemalan colleagues told me about a patient who had a gynecological surgery at a jornada, during which the surgeon unwittingly cut through cancerous tissue. The patient had never had a Pap smear, no tissue was analyzed before the operation, and none of the removed tissues were retained for analysis after the surgery. The Guatemalan doctors pointed out that such a patient should not have been operated on, that the North American surgeon would never have operated like this in North America without the pre- and postoperative analyses, and that the operation hastened the patient's death.

This haunting story highlights one of the conflicts facing surgical missions: as they frequently operated outside of a fully functioning clinic or medical unit, their resources were limited. At the time of the fateful surgery, the resources available to the jornada would have been on par with what was available in other clinics or the hospital in that region. Yet, Teresa grew frustrated that, as the medical infrastructure improved in Sololá, jornadas' management of surgery did not necessarily follow suit. While she herself had operated for years without access to "pathology and pre-ops labs," now that those were available, she no longer felt that it was "right" do so. She described to me her frustration with jornadas' reluctance to change:

> These guys would come in and act like they were on top of the mountain and there were no services available. . . . We had a big discussion with them. . . . I said, "Look, you guys. You think you're out in the wild, but right here in Sololá, by now, we have a CT scanner. We have an X-ray—what is it—clinic or whatever. We have a full lab, totally certified. We have blood transfusions." I mean, really Sololá and the private sector has evolved. . . . I told Finn, "This has got to stop. These guys have got to do things the right way." But okay, that's my worst critique [of STMMs].

In this quote, Teresa brings to the fore the importance of contexts that are changing through time to situated judgments. As she says, at one time, the medical infrastructure in Sololá was so impoverished that she felt it would be better to do surgery with the limited information available than not to do it at all. But, as the context changed and medical infrastructure improved, Teresa's judgment regarding what was "the right way" changed. While it was right to perform surgeries without access to laboratory and other exams when none were available, she viewed it as wrong to do so when they were available. The problem was that the volunteers did not keep up with the contextual changes; they presumed what was acceptable instead of trying to keep apprised of how things transformed through time, arguably to the jeopardy of their patients.

Both Teresa and her fellow STMM surgeon volunteers make judgments on whether to operate on a patient in the context of a jornada. However, Teresa's situated judgments foreground context, whereas other STMM volunteers presume a static situation based on their ideas of place that may not reflect the realities of health care in Guatemala. In her remarks, Teresa critiques her colleagues for operating on patients with insufficient preparation. Teresa's action is situated in relation to contextual knowledge about the particular medical landscape in Sololá at a particular moment in time, as she contends. Yet, during her interview, Teresa indicated that jornadas in Sololá seemed to disregard this contextual and temporal point. Teresa tried to convince jornadas to "do things the right way," and she spoke with each jornada she worked with to let it know what resources were available. Nevertheless, jornadas continued to practice without integrating new, available resources, a decision that Teresa criticized but that seems consonant with the idea that Sololá is more of a backdrop than an active influence on what goes on at a jornada.

The example of the patient with undetected cancer highlights the moral peril of operating at a jornada. Indeed, as we can see from Teresa's comments, judging when to operate should be the moral foundation of STMMs. Nevertheless, as Teresa indicates and as I witnessed, within jornadas, volunteers displayed what seemed to be insufficient discomfort with these particular decisions. Despite Teresa's doubts regarding what should be happening and what was happening, volunteers seemed relatively confident that these were morally good choices, leading to good outcomes for patients.[10] How is this confidence possible?

Another volunteer, Hazel, was also unsettled by her fellow volunteers' confidence that carrying out their professional roles in a jornada necessarily constituted good actions. Hazel was a clinician who had volunteered for many years locally with different organizations, including Doctors Without Borders, in her Canadian city. Hazel explained that volunteering was an important part of her life because it had helped her cope with a difficult divorce; during that time, she said, "I got a lot of help from my friends." For her, volunteering was a way "to give back to society," notably echoing sentiments discussed earlier regarding the particular and personal nature of the reasons for engaging in global health work.

Hazel was adventurous and wanted to try working abroad but could not afford the nine-month commitment with Doctors Without Borders. Eventually she heard about a mission opportunity through her church, and she completed two different missions in sub-Saharan African countries. Subsequently, her colleagues recommended that she work with a different organization that went to Guatemala, and she signed up.

Hazel echoed the idea that just going on a mission and slotting into your professional role did not guarantee that the actions you took would do good. Indeed, she began her interview by telling me that she had seen colleagues go on missions without accomplishing much. Illustrating this, she said, "These groups go there, and it's just like a holiday. They don't do anything. . . . It all depends . . . on the individual." When Hazel said that it "depends on the individual," she meant that the volunteers have to make a specific effort to ensure that their actions would have a positive impact; without that extra effort, merely volunteering on these missions is not necessarily a morally good act. She said, "I know it's a lot of work if you want to make a difference in someone's life. It's not that easy. [It's about] whether you really want to go that extra mile." For Hazel, the "extra mile" involved taking in the context, going out of your way to talk to people (not just patients), and then "seeing what they need."

Notably, Hazel had several stories from multiple different missions emphasizing her judgment that she had to take not only medical action but also nonmedical action if she wanted her mission work to build her ethical life. For instance, during one mission in Guatemala, Hazel treated a man who had been injured in an industrial accident. Four of his coworkers had died, and though he and another coworker survived, he was left paraplegic. When Hazel first visited him, she was humbled by his living conditions. She described the setting for me: "When we first met him, he was full of bedsores from top to bottom. They gave him one year to live. There were flies everywhere. You should have seen where he stayed. He had a gap—between the roof and the walls, a big gap—so in the winter, it's cold. In the summer, it's hot. There are flies. It's not even a house. It's a shack. That's where he lived." He was married with two children, but he was now unable to work, leaving the family unable to care for him or themselves. Hazel decided to become a sponsor for the family and committed herself to making sure their conditions improved. Her first step was to find sustained financial support for the family by getting twelve of her friends to commit to giving her ten dollars a month. "This is how I put it to my friends for the $120 every year. Every year. I say, 'If you buy a cup of Starbucks coffee, it's two-something. It's ten dollars a month, I'm asking you. That's just three cups of coffee. Can you do it?'" She secured an arrangement with an NGO in Guatemala that could take her friends' donations and distribute the entire amount only to this family. She then used her networks to get donations of medical equipment that could improve the man's day-to-day struggle with mobility. Two years later, she returned to see him, and he only had one bedsore and was doing well; his family was also thriving. At the time of the interview, many years after first meeting this man, she was still supporting the family. This example illustrates Hazel's contention that "the individual" is the one who needs to figure out how whether to "do anything" in specific circumstances. In her view, flying to Guatemala with a group and treating the man's bedsores was abrogating her moral responsibility; for her to feel like she was doing something good, she needed to make a sustainable difference in his life and in all the lives that she touched.

While both Hazel and Teresa want to improve conditions for their communities, each judged that fulfilling their medical roles in a faraway land was insufficient to do this. Hazel's story emphasizes that she could not possibly have foretold what she needed to do to fulfill her own moral obligations before she went to Guatemala. Teresa echoed a similar sentiment, but to it she added time. She told me that her judgments regarding what she could and should change had altered as more time passed. As Teresa put it, "I always wanted to make things a little bit better, but I really agree with Finn. I think change has to come from the people. You can't force it." In her analysis, her desire to "cure the world" does not sufficiently specify what she has to do on an everyday level to "make things a little better."

While Teresa's desire to "make things better" might be a constant ethical imperative in her life, her quote makes clear that situated judgments respond to the changes in the context in which she is working. We see both new relationships blossom and old ones foreclose. We also see changes in what is possible—while Finn and Teresa spent most of their time during the civil war "making things better" one surgery at a time, the end of the war created new opportunities in Sololá. We can understand Finn and Teresa's participation in jornadas as part of this constant effort to judge how they can make a difference within each particular context.

## DIY Global Health, Situated Judgment, and Visceral Ethics

Looking at the experience of someone who had extensive global health practice in Sololá highlights the importance of context to making situated judgments of actions. It also calls into question moral judgments that are made without contextual considerations. Indeed, the examples from this chapter shift us from one frame, in which a volunteer merely takes action (e.g., goes to a jornada; once there, does surgery), to an alternate frame, in which this truncated experience places the volunteer in moral peril. Furthermore, this shift highlights how, in the absence of contextual considerations, visceral ethics—that is, judgments based on gut feelings—replace situated judgments.

While working for an STMM is undoubtedly part of a volunteer's ethical life, participating in DIY global health action does not automatically contribute to a good life. Teresa's and Hazel's narratives show us that, even while living a life aimed to create positive change for others, they judged their actions as good—or not—based on the outcomes of those actions. Their narratives speak to the fact that blanket judgments about global health action being good (or bad) are misleading; furthermore, it is impossible to make blanket judgments about *one's own* global health action as good (or bad).

I suggest that volunteers' confidence in their actions as constituting good work is inspired by affect. Our gut feelings about the work that we do *stands in* for situated judgments.[11] Indeed, visceral ethics helps explain the surprising confidence that I myself and other volunteers had when engaging in our activities. As we saw earlier, these gut feelings can even outweigh concrete details, like available medical resources, which might militate against good patient outcomes.

This chapter also addresses why visceral ethics can be so tightly bound to global health practice. Indeed, when practitioners work in places where they lack an understanding of context, they are able to fill in the gaps with a sense of moral action in the absence of necessary situated judgments. This option typically is not available in a home country, where practitioners are working within a familiar context.

In chapter 5, I take up these themes. I further consider how this lack of knowing what we have done in DIY global health work opens the door for visceral ethics to be the primary barometer of what happens at jornadas. Not only is a sufficient rendering of context and, therefore, situated judgment missing, but volunteers also lack sufficient information about patient outcomes to evaluate specific impacts of their actions, let alone long-term residual effects of STMMs. I argue that this lack of information colludes with volunteers' intentions to lead ethical lives, resulting in volunteers' reliance on their gut feelings to make sense of the ethical nature of their work.

5

# Where There Is No Doctor

*Ethical Lives in the Absence of Feedback*

The title of this chapter is a play on the title of a popular book published by Hesperian Health Guides, *Where There Is No Doctor* (Werner, Thuman, & Maxwell, 2017). Before the internet, *Where There Is No Doctor* was often found in the suitcases of global health workers traveling from the North to places like Guatemala. The title of this chapter aims to connect us to the familiar narrative that STMMs go where there is no doctor to provide medical care, despite the fact that this is frequently not true, as is the case in Sololá.[1] For STMMs, locations marked by an absence of care are fundamental to "ideas of place," discussed in the introduction.

This chapter digs more deeply into the relationship between ideas of place and visceral ethics. More specifically, it looks at how decontextualization strips away the sources of feedback needed to judge moral action. I argue in this chapter that in the absence of feedback, volunteers judge the ways in which they deploy their professional knowledge to determine the moral nature of their global health action. The tight focus on professional frames and lack of contextual feedback creates a gut confidence that, even in unsettling circumstances, the action taken was good.

Orlando, a Guatemalan doctor who worked for the Ministry of Health, pointed out a potential disconnect in using jornada work to build an ethical life. Everyone likes to help others, he said, and donating their time to a jornada makes volunteers feel good. However, he thought that it was a major problem that people who volunteered in jornadas did not have the opportunity to see the results of their work. They could not know if what they did really benefited anyone. As he said, "It might be that [jornada work] was beneficial, or it might be that there was a complication and maybe [the patient] died a month later, but [the volunteer] still feels good" (translation by author). Orlando's comment suggests that what happens to the patient in the aftermath of jornada care should inform how those volunteers judge their work. If not, volunteers' judgments of their own moral actions are seriously truncated as they remain predicated only on how they spend their own time.

Despite the thousands of medical missions happening every year, there is a paucity of attempts to document patient outcomes, even among surgical STMMs, where knowledge regarding mid- to long-term patient outcomes would be particularly important.[2] Indeed, the evaluation of medical missions remain problematically centered on prospective accounting of patient satisfaction and delivery of care (Berry, 2014; Wilson, 2021). Also telling is the state of MESH terms for medical missions. MESH terms are the standardized subject headings that power Medline/PubMed, the most important search engine for accessing biomedical research. The MESH term "medical missions" was introduced in 2019, yet as of writing this, there is no subheading related to medical outcomes, which indicates how underdeveloped this literature is. This dearth of documentation not only points to an absence of information regarding mid- or long-term patient outcomes but also hints at an absence of abiding interest in pursuing questions about patient outcomes more broadly.

This is surprising for me given how uncertain care regimes are at a jornada in comparison to the care that volunteers provide in their home countries. We saw a glimpse of this earlier regarding the scarcity of night nurses in the hospital ward. Indeed, in North America, the health care infrastructure creates a routine system of care that is relatively reliable. This system of care means that physicians are required to perform only their specific roles and can thus rely on others to complete treatment plans. Yet, care provision at a jornada can be less reliable. Often, the care provided by an STMM is disconnected from other sources of care. Meanwhile, jornada care incorporates few accountability and workflow measures; as a result, providers rarely know what happens to their patients after they see them, let alone remain responsible for continued follow-up attention. Moreover, as depicted in these accounts, patients seeking public or private follow-up care in Guatemala can face myriad issues because they usually lack Spanish-language medical records, (records of) lab results or preoperative exams, and the ability to contact STMM doctors to debrief their Guatemalan physicians. In interviews, volunteers repeatedly pointed to this lack of follow-up care as trouble-some from a medical perspective.

Thus, we return to the question that haunted our discussion of situated judgments and that drives this chapter: How do volunteers build ethical lives in the absence of the information that they need to evaluate the morality of their actions? The answer that emerged from my data is that they fixate on what they *do* know. This chapter shows how, in the absence of necessary contextual knowledge, volunteers judge whether their actions are moral by relying on their own professional knowledge. As we have seen, a disregard for context erases important information about where STMMs take place. As hinted in the title of the chapter and as Orlando points out, the feedback that would illuminate the consequences of action (i.e., what happened to patients treated) is unavailable. Yet, in the spaces of these absences, STMM volunteers' understandings of their own choices to join jornadas and their own professional conduct while there reverberate. Volunteers thus come to rely heavily on a professional lens to judge action as moral. Professional confidence can override gut doubt, causing volunteers to feel good about their actions, regardless of what they might or might not understand about their long-term effects on patients or the health systems where they work.

To illustrate how volunteers rely on professional knowledge to substantiate the moral nature of their actions, I review one particular clinical encounter that occurred during the last day of a weeklong short-term medical mission. The case involved four different volunteers, including me. This reflection is substantiated by my field notes and by conversations that I had with each volunteer after I returned to Canada. It illustrates how we, as volunteers, had inadequate information about the local milieu and the effects of our work. Reviewing this case also helps highlight the ways in which we process these situations; each of us involved in this encounter drew on our own past professional experiences to make sense of what happened. Ultimately, the security (or, in my case, insecurity) that those professional positions generated produced a gut feeling within each of us, viscerally substantiating or undermining our understandings of our actions as moral.

## An Encounter with Claudia

Claudia was seventeen years old, married, and pregnant for the first time. She lived in the nearby predominantly K'iche' Maya city of Nahualá and dressed in a *huipil* and *corte*.[3] Claudia told us that she came to the jornada because senior women in her family had told her that she should go and get the baby scanned. Her family members were waiting outside the gate while she came in the clinic. I was in the room serving as a translator, working with a clinician, Heather. Claudia was visibly pregnant. When I asked her why she was there, she said that she did not want vitamins or anything else; she only wanted to see the baby. She sat on the examination bed, and, while Heather took her history, I translated. When the sonographer, Stephanie, arrived, she put the transducer on Claudia's abdomen to examine the baby. But a moment later, Stephanie immediately stopped the ultrasound and said that we needed to move to a darker room so that she could see the screen better. As soon as Stephanie said we needed to move, Claudia asked if the baby was okay. I said that they did not know yet because they could not see the screen of the machine in the bright room. I explained to Claudia that we had to move to a room without a window, and we waited tensely while a new location was found. After about five minutes, we settled into a new exam room and began the process again. Stephanie scanned Claudia's abdomen, showing her the baby on the screen as we listened to the heartbeat. As Stephanie said that we needed to wait for another clinician to come who would speak with Claudia about her baby's health, I translated the information to Claudia. The incoming clinician would speak Spanish and be able to answer all of Claudia's questions.

While it was not clear to me at the time, Stephanie noticed in the original scan that the baby did not have a brain. Asking to change rooms was a stall tactic. While looking for a different room, she went to find Ana, a clinician fluent in Spanish, to confirm the diagnosis and speak directly to Claudia.

When Ana came in, she looked at the scan and delivered the news. She told Claudia that the baby was not healthy, that the baby might not be born alive, and that if it was born alive, it would not live for very long. Ana told Claudia that, because of this condition, it was important for Claudia to deliver in the hospital. She emphasized that it was not

Claudia's fault and that sometimes this just happens. Ana then asked if Claudia had any questions, and Claudia said no. Ana left, and Heather tried to reach out to Claudia, while I translated. Heather asked if Claudia wanted some prenatal vitamins for her health, to which Claudia said no. Heather then told Claudia that this sort of pregnancy would probably never happen to her again. Heather asked Claudia if there was anyone outside whom Claudia might want us to get, to perhaps explain the situation to them. Again, Claudia declined. I wrote in my field notes that, though Claudia sat on the examination bed smiling at us the entire time, it was obvious to me that she was eager to leave. The smile felt like a performance, maybe to placate our concerns by masking her own emotions. When Heather ran out of questions and the consultation came to an end, Claudia quickly got up and left the facility.

When I spoke to Heather nine months later, she mentioned our encounter with Claudia before I even had a chance to ask her about it. Heather used Claudia's case as an example to explain to me why she would want to have better cultural knowledge and communication skills if she were to volunteer for another mission. By the time Claudia had come into the exam room, we had already seen a few pregnant women throughout the jornada. Heather had conducted prenatal checkups with each of them and found nothing concerning. Heather told me that Claudia probably had no idea that anything was wrong because the baby was probably still moving and because, as Heather put it, "she was measuring well," meaning that her uterus was a good size for how far along she was in her pregnancy. The lack of signs of concern and the relative rarity of Claudia's condition meant that when Stephanie started the scan, Heather said that no one, not the clinicians or Claudia, was expecting to find this anomaly.

Heather felt cast adrift because so many of her skills were attenuated due to the language barrier between herself and her client. She began to feel this acutely when Stephanie did the original scan. She told me, "I remember doing our sono and then seeing the baby, and the baby did not look good. . . . There was a moment like, how to even communicate this to her? Because we do have a language barrier." Normally in a case like this, Heather would be the one to "explain what was going on," but in this case, all she could do was watch Ana talk to Claudia. Though she could not understand what was being said, Heather told me she was "watching the patient or watching her nonverbal [body language]":

> It just didn't look like [Claudia] totally had a really good understanding of what happened. . . . It was her eyes. . . . It almost felt like there was a blank look—not like an understanding, not an emotion, more just like flat. And really she didn't ask any questions either, which is unusual when somebody tells you something like that. You know, it was more—she was so quiet. You know, normally the patient might be quiet, but they're going to have questions. They might be crying, whatever, but usually there's just more conversation, and she was so still. There wasn't really much from her at all.

Heather was not satisfied that the patient was okay, but she was "just really feeling kind of at a loss as to what to do."

To help me understand her sense of unease in Claudia's case, Heather started to compare what happened at the jornada with what would have happened to this kind of case in North America. In her practice, Heather would have taken the client directly to the labor and delivery unit to see a perinatologist. Not only would Heather have remained with the client, but she also would have brought in the client's chosen "support person." The perinatologist would have then reviewed everything that was known about the case with the client and their support person so that they could understand "exactly what that means at this moment in time for her pregnancy and what would happen." The client would then be counseled on her options, including what would happen if she decided to induce versus carry the baby to term, making sure she understood that there was no chance that the baby would survive. Heather pointed out that this whole encounter of explaining, listening, and talking was critical and that she would not be satisfied until she knew that the client and her support person understood everything and had asked sufficient questions. Finally, she would make sure that the client was referred to a bereavement group and had a social/emotional support plan. Heather stressed that "even if she wasn't quite interested [in counseling] at this point, . . . they follow her to make sure, because this is someone who would be at huge risk for postpartum depression."

Obviously, none of these resources were available at the jornada, and Heather wondered if we should have taken Claudia then to the nearest hospital. Heather would have felt good about this decision if she were in North America, but in Guatemala, she did not know what was right. Would Claudia or her family be comfortable relying on the biomedical care provided at the hospital? Heather worried that she could not even be certain that sending someone to the hospital or accompanying them there was the right thing to do because it might be "outside their culture." She said, "It would be really nice to know who, . . . like culturally— who we could talk to to make sure [Claudia] was okay. Or is that even appropriate?" She also lamented the lack of "integrat[ion]" of her work at the jornada with the wider Guatemalan health system, be it among formal or informal providers. She had an idea of what sorts of services might be good for Claudia to access, but she had no idea if or where those types of services were available in Guatemala. This made it even more difficult for Heather to ascertain what to tell Claudia.

Once Claudia received the news, Heather said that it was "like it was going in slow motion, and it was surreal that this was actually even happening." As Heather recounts, the next thing we knew, "Claudia kind of just got up and left." Heather still felt that something had been "off" in the interaction. Looking back, she guessed that Claudia probably was not going to say anything to her family waiting outside for her. Heather said, "[I] almost wanted to chase after her, but what was I going to say to her in English?" again reaffirming her original point that she wanted to develop better language skills before doing another jornada.

We spent some time talking about what happened and if we could have done anything differently. In the end, Heather did not think she would have changed what we did. Her major takeaways concerned the need to improve her local language skills and the need for the jornada to become more integrated into the health care system so that cases could be directed appropriately. She also mused about the STMM structure and how it complicated cases like this: "Another drawback, I guess, [is] not to go back to where we were at." Heather is referring to the fact that, once volunteers for missions leave, they typically never return to the mission site and never see the patients again. Heather continued with this thought: "It's probably a drawback of a short-term mission in the sense that you don't have the follow-through. You don't know what ends up happening. Because most of us like to know what happens to our patients." Without any sort of feedback, it was impossible to know what had happened to Claudia after she left us.

Charles Salmen et al.'s (2022) intervention into the science of working in the global health domain to improve outcomes provides some useful concepts that help explain how Heather filled in the gaps to understand the encounter with Claudia. The authors draw on a phenomenon called the "illusion of control" from social psychology to explain "the global health community['s] . . . remarkable level of self-assurance" that making studies and interventions more "rigorous" will help meet global health challenges (Salmen et al., 2022:4008). The illusion of control refers to the idea that individuals draw on *skill cues* and consequently overestimate their control over random events. Skill cues are any cues that relate back to an individual's "exercise of expertise" (Salmen et al., 2022:4008).[4] Salmen et al. put forth the idea that we gravitate toward our own areas of expertise to make sense of the randomness or lack of control that global health work presents. For example, Heather expresses doubts about her current preparedness and dissatisfaction regarding her lack of ability to follow up with Claudia. Nevertheless, it was her evaluation of her own professional conduct that she used to judge what happened. Heather anchored this uncertain encounter in areas of her own expertise. Narrowing the domain of evaluation so that it cleaves closely to her professional capacity allows her to assure herself that she did her best.[5]

This example helps bring to the fore how, in the absence of feedback, reliance on professional expertise can encourage gut confidence in the moral valence of action. Following Salmen et al. (2022), Heather relies on certain parts of the encounter—that is, the parts relating to her own professional conduct—as key to judging her action. Because she is so capable, relying on a professional evaluation gives her confidence in her action. Yet, her confidence is not anchored in what happens in the context of Sololá. Heather was explicit regarding her lack of understanding of who and what was available in the health system and that this gap precluded her from being able to make any referrals. When all is said and done, as Orlando points out, her confidence remained unchallenged: what might or might not happen to Claudia in the wake of our consultation cannot figure into how Heather comes to see her action as moral (or not).[6] Because of the design of short-term medical missions, the medical staff that treated Claudia will never receive feedback about what happened to her.

Stephanie's account of the case further conveys how skill cues and professional expertise connect to volunteers' judgments of jornada work as moral action. Stephanie told me that she did not go on the jornada with the intention of scanning pregnant women but rather to use imaging to help with surgery patients. Nevertheless, Claudia's case was the third and last prenatal ultrasound that she had done. The other two had been a source of joy, getting to show mothers their babies and letting them hear the fetal heartbeats. Stephanie described to me what she remembered about the encounter with Claudia:

> I set down the transducer, and the first thing I saw was that there was polyhydramnios, which is too much fluid around the baby. Then the next—I started looking at the rest of the baby, and the baby had anencephaly. Anencephaly is when they don't have a head or a brain. They have a face. Then I looked at the baby's heart, and it had an abnormal heart. With all those findings, it was probably a trisomy 13, which is not compatible with life. She was just—before I even scanned her again, she was this . . . young girl, very sweet, just coming in, I think, to see her baby. That was the only reason; she wasn't having any other complications.

This last point, that Stephanie was not scanning Claudia for diagnostic information but rather to let her "see her baby," was important to Stephanie as she did not know enough about Sololá and the people who live there to say that this was necessarily a sufficient purpose. Perhaps because her career was so tightly focused on the use of technology in medicine, Stephanie's reflection on Claudia's case cleaved closely to the role of technology in medical missions. She believed that technology was a powerful tool when applied with purpose but that it was important to be clear about what that purpose was. She explained this to me by saying,

> If they're pregnant and they have a question about the pregnancy, for us to do an ultrasound on them [is beneficial], because there's things that could be sort of lifesaving to the mom, too. Like, what if the baby's not alive,

and she hasn't miscarried? . . . I just think that we do just sort of need to be careful in how much we're doing. . . . I don't know enough about the Mayan culture yet. I don't know if it's something that we should advertise, like, "Please come let us see your baby," kind of thing informational-wise to their population."

We can see from this quote that, though Stephanie is trained in imaging, she conceptualizes her work as part of a larger system of care. While she did not shun the idea of seeing a woman's baby just for fun, she worried about the decision to provide scans for her clients at the jornada because of potential "cultural" differences. In unpacking what this meant to her, Stephanie reflected on Claudia's case: "Culturally, when the baby was born, I worried, 'Would [Claudia] be shunned from her village? Would they think it was something that she did?'" She explained to me about her practice, "I always tell my patients . . . 'knowledge is power,' that you have to decide how much knowledge you want as a family." In this case, she was unable to predict the reactions of others to the news because she lacked an understanding of what was appropriate and because her patient did not offer any meaningful feedback about how to proceed. Because of that, this case worried her. She asked me, "Was it really a good thing that she found . . . out [that her baby was going to die]?" Like Heather, Stephanie felt too unfamiliar with the context to answer her question.

Part of Stephanie's doubt had to do with Claudia's reaction to the news. Stephanie emphasized that after receiving the diagnosis, Claudia was "very stoic about it and then didn't have anybody there with her and just seemed to sort of want to leave": "Even though we gave her the information, [there were] essentially no questions asked on her part." While Stephanie had seen other patients "go into shock" when they received "bad news," she did not usually worry about that as much as she did in this case. She explained, "My patients are able to call back to my office and say, 'All right, I'm ready to hear what you have to say now about this. Can we talk about it? I need this information,' or, 'I'm really struggling with this. I'm so sad. I don't know how to handle it. I need somebody to talk to.' Then we also will—we'll literally spend up to two hours with some patients counseling them on the bad news." In this case, though, she knew that it would not happen. Once Claudia left the room, we would never hear from or see her again. This was particularly difficult for Stephanie, who told me, "I just broke down and cried because I wanted to counsel her more. I wanted her to stay there, and I wanted her to have time to absorb what was going on. That wasn't the case. Those were my own wants."

Like Heather, Stephanie found Claudia's case difficult to deal with, and she unpacked those difficulties in relation to her own professional role. While Stephanie was not worried about her technical ability to conduct an ultrasound or read the visual output correctly, she was worried about the larger role of technology in the jornada. She was not used to operating in circumstances in which the mandate of her role was unclear. Indeed, what gave her doubt was that there was no system in place at the jornada that governed the purpose of ultrasounds. She just found herself doing a prenatal scan because she was present and able.

Juxtaposing Stephanie's and Heather's responses helps clarify the importance of skill cues to volunteers' judgments of what happened. In both situations, volunteers seem to be making sense of the interaction by comparing it to more typical interactions that they have in their own practices in North America. Heather was concerned about not speaking the same language because it made her unable to get an accurate pulse on the situation. This was not something she typically encountered in her work. While Stephanie also wished that Claudia had stayed and talked, she focused on Claudia's right to choose to leave. It was harder for Stephanie to accept the lack of clear mandate around imaging; thus, she questioned her reasons for performing the scan.

Ana, the Spanish-speaking doctor whom Stephanie fetched, also drew on skill cues to make sense of what had happened with Claudia. Yet, unlike the other two, Ana's analysis of the case emphasized how standard the encounter was. The first thing that she remembered was Stephanie being really upset. "I remember Stephanie coming over in tears because she diagnosed it. It was an anencephalic baby, I think is what it was, which is when the baby has no cranium on the top of the head. That's a pretty lethal anomaly. . . . I went in, and I confirmed the diagnosis. Then, we just had a very straightforward conversation with the patient about what the baby had, to the best of my ability, in laymen's terms." While Ana referenced Claudia's blank affect and lack of questions, her frame was tightly cleaved to the diagnosis and what the patient needed to know about it. Ana felt that "it was certainly—obviously, less than ideal": "I think, from the physician perspective, it makes sense for her to know. We were able to give her some very concrete instructions about what to do." Ana went over a lot of the potential complications that can result from this type of pregnancy, for example, that sometimes these babies do not trigger labor and that they can be breech, so Ana advised her to deliver in the hospital. She also told Claudia that she could, however, deliver the baby vaginally and did not need a scheduled Caesarean section. From Ana's perspective, much of what transpired in that interaction was similar to what would have happened in North America. As she put, "It's pretty much standard to take a look at any baby, to do an anatomy check halfway through the pregnancy." When she considered what happened after she confirmed the diagnosis, Ana said, "Claudia got bad news. I'm not sure that the quiet reaction would've been any different in the States. When people go through those five stages of grief, she may have just gone straight into stun mode and maybe a little bit of denial." In short, Ana emphasized how this interaction was routine for her as it mirrored encounters with patients in the United States.

As the fourth volunteer who was with Claudia, I also turned to skill cues to make sense of the situation. Though the other three found skill cues in the clinical aspects of the care, I was more attentive to the social dynamics of care. Medical anthropologists tend to be wary of approaches that center the individual (as biomedical, clinical care tends to do) without considering the influence of wider structures (Borovoy & Hine, 2008; Scheper-Hughes & Lock, 1987). This issue has been particularly present in policies and programs aimed at women's reproductive health—for example, interventions aimed at getting individual sex workers to use condoms in contexts where clients do not want to use condoms (Khalid & Martin, 2019; Wojcicki & Malala, 2001). Approaches to women's pregnancy and family planning that center individual women have tended to encode assumptions prevalent in North American middle- and upper-class (White) feminist discourse that emphasize women's autonomy and "choice" as the center of good care and improved health outcomes (Chi et al., 2011; Mumtaz & Salway, 2009). My earlier work in Sololá contrasted the focus on individual women in interventions to improve maternal survival with the inherently intersubjective process of pregnancy and reproduction in a Kaqchikel Maya region where I lived and worked. A choice-focused narrative positions a woman as a gatekeeper, responsible for deciding what she wants in her pregnancy and who will be involved in supporting her. It centers her by making the pregnancy about her. Importantly, pregnancy in the Kaqchikel area where I lived had been a "kinning" event that could bind members of families more closely together (Berry, 2010). The first birth was particularly important for new daughters-in-law joining their husband's family. Many different actors had assigned roles to play in bringing the baby into the world, for example, contracting a midwife, paying the midwife, supporting the woman in labor, and deciding when and if there was a problem. The mother did not selectively choose who would be involved in caring for her. In sum, in the region of Sololá where I lived, understanding pregnancy, especially a first pregnancy, through this relational lens was more important for a woman's long-term well-being than was the individual lens that is so typical to biomedicine.

Although Claudia came from a vastly different context than the one with which I was familiar (e.g., she was K'iche', not Kaqchikel; she was also from a densely populated periurban area, not a village), it was nonetheless still my professional knowledge that sprang forward and undergirded my response. My immediate concern was that we had arranged the provision of care in a manner that undercut Claudia's web of support. Like many clinical environments, we had limited space and wanted to prioritize accommodating patients. This frequently meant that the numerous family members who often accompanied a patient would wait outside the gate, and the patient came in to see the clinician. While this may be an effective strategy for clinical treatment, medical anthropologists have long pointed out the disconnect between organizing care provision around treatment of patients and the more complex family dynamics that often determine responsibility and processes around medical decision-making (Cohen, 1998; Foley, 2008; Janzen, 1978; Unnithan & Kasstan, 2021). I had seen this dynamic in action when it came to decision-making around pregnancy. For example, women I had interviewed for my dissertation research frequently pinned the responsibility of deciding to go to the hospital for birthing issues on their midwife, mother, mother-in-law, husband, or some combination of those. Younger women were particularly unlikely to see themselves as responsible for making that decision. At just seventeen years of age and experiencing her first pregnancy, Claudia was certainly part of the younger demographic. The distributions of responsibility that occurred around pregnancy had an intended benefit of making sure that a woman did not have to shoulder particularly weighty burdens by herself. She could depend on her elders to take on the charge of determining a recommended course of action, because they have more lived experience and typically desired the best outcomes for her. (Indeed, Claudia had told us that her elders advised her to come and have the fetus imaged.) In retrospect, I was worried that pulling Claudia off on her own and giving her a diagnosis was unfair, and that worry sat in my gut when I thought about Claudia. We were burdening her while removing her support people, who were supposed to be handling this sort of situation.

Our encounter with Claudia also recalled another situation that had played out decades ago when I was first starting my fieldwork in the health district. At that time, Pap smears were not widely available and, when ordered at the public hospital, had to be sent to a laboratory in Guatemala City. At the beginning of the 2000s, a new, low-tech method for the identification and treatment of irregular cervical cells began to be promoted for primary care in low-income settings (Belinson et al., 2001). Rather than having to send a cell sample to a lab, trained providers could now use acetic acid to stain cervical tissue, conduct a visual inspection of the cervix, and freeze or burn off any suspect cells. In Guatemala, this method was first deployed by a number of NGOs that were involved in reproductive health (Chary & Rohloff, 2014). One NGO decided to create a mobile screening unit, which came to the district where I lived. A Ministry of Health employee who worked in the district told me that the campaign ended poorly. While looking for irregular cells, they found a woman a few villages over who had been diagnosed with cervical cancer. The NGO gave her the information that she had cancer, but there was no treatment available to her. The person recounting this story to me said that people in the village had found this very upsetting—it was cruel to tell someone that they were going to die imminently. The social anthropologist Susan Reynolds Whyte (2002) writes extensively about this conundrum with reference to HIV diagnosis in an era before antiretroviral drugs were available to control the virus. She argues that receiving a diagnosis of HIV was akin to killing people's hope. As long as the diagnosis was uncertain, there was always a possibility that a patient or loved one could get better. Once the diagnosis was delivered, all hope was lost. I was troubled by the parallels between Claudia's case and these examples. I worried that it was equally cruel to tell a young woman who was seemingly happy and worry-free in her first pregnancy that her baby was not healthy.

Like Luz's case that begins this book, Claudia's case haunted me. While memories of Antonia's tumor lying in a tub while she sat transformed, or a child being gifted sight, invigorated me, remembering when Ana delivered the news to Claudia about her baby tempered my enthusiasm. As the months passed, I realized that I wanted to reconnect with three other volunteers with whom I had worked on Claudia's case, to learn what they remembered and how they felt about it. As highlighted in these pages, while Ana's perspective of her own obligations to Claudia were straightforward, both Heather and Stephanie wrangled with the complexity of this case. Regardless, Claudia's case did not make either feel any less certain that volunteering at an STMM contributed to building their ethical lives.

I was surprised that this case did not change Heather's and Stephanie's opinions about medical missions. In my conversation with Heather, I brought up my own discomfort from a moral perspective about dumping potentially unactionable, heart-wrenching information on Claudia when we would have no future contact with her. "It is hard to get my head around not telling her," Heather said. She made the point that, even if Claudia "hadn't come in that day, she would have had a stillborn baby." Claudia might not have understood everything that we told her, but from Heather's perspective, a seed of acknowledgment had been planted. Heather had seen many families go through pregnancies that ended with undesired outcomes; she felt that knowing can bring acceptance. Although Heather acknowledged that there was a possibility that we had "failed" Claudia, the outcome of this case did not change her opinion on the ethical value of jornadas. Even if we had failed Claudia, Heather saw it as an opportunity for learning and improvement.

After speaking with Heather, Ana, and Stephanie, I was surprised to find that my doubts about our actions in this case lingered. I was not reassured by my own gut that we had done the right thing. Going back over their narratives, I realized how buttressed each was by (different) standards of care that undergirded their judgment and directed them how to act. Fitting this case into a medical frame gave them confidence and provided them some certainty in a sea of unknown. Because I lack that medical frame and drew on a different (and perhaps more skeptical) professional narrative, I could not feel confident. Moreover, while the actions that we had taken perhaps met rigorous standards of practice, what we did inside the clinic did not address the fundamental point of why we were there at all. We were volunteers. We had made the choice to insert ourselves into patients' lives on the basis of the supposition that we would be helpful. We were leaving that week. Claiming the authority and responsibility to make important medical interventions in people's lives in such a time-limited way felt morally perilous. Nonetheless, it was clear that we had all found our own ways to process what had occurred, although we would never actually learn what happened to Claudia.

## Visceral Ethics: Moral Action in Ideas of Place

In this chapter, Claudia's example highlights how visceral ethics functions to create confidence and even certainty in volunteering, despite murky situations. Notably, volunteers rarely find out what happens to patients. Because of this, judgments of our own actions are often unmoored from the actual consequences of these actions. The problem in this arrangement, as Orlando so poignantly points out, is that volunteers can return home still feeling good about our work, even if we caused something bad to happen. In the absence of contextual feedback, confidence in one's own professional knowledge comes to occupy an important role in rendering one's own actions as moral. Confidence that caring for patients at an STMM was good moral action is easy when everything seems to be going right. If things go wrong, confidence is frequently generated from volunteers' gut feelings that they did the best they could professionally in the given circumstances.

What makes it possible to build an ethical life in this way? I opened this chapter by articulating the narrative that STMMs unfold in places where there is no health care available for the people who live there. The narrative creates an allure: Who would not want to step in to help those who have no help? But this narrative is also part of a constructed idea of place. One of the consequences of this idea of place is that it interrupts volunteers' interest in being meaningfully attached to the context in which they work. We saw this in chapter 4 when Teresa pointed out how difficult it was to get STMMs to plug into medical resources that were available in Sololá. We further see this with Claudia's example. Heather pinpointed her frustration at not knowing what (if any) referrals she could make. Claudia's consultation highlighted the importance of contextual factors to a clear understanding of how we could have best handled this case (e.g., informing family, plugging her into follow-up care). Yet ultimately, researching context so that other volunteers might not face such an unsettling consultation does not fit into the ephemeral nature of DIY global health. Though Claudia's consultation galvanized both Heather and Stephanie to consider reforms, these reforms would exist within the jornada—disconnected to place. In short, there is a notable lack of curiosity or attentiveness to context. Instead, volunteers' analyses represent the jornada as an integrated whole and Sololá as a decontextualized, peripheral backdrop.

Ideas of place are paramount to making STMMs available to volunteers to build their ethical lives. An idea of place decouples the actions that a volunteer takes from actual places and actual consequences. Kevin Sykes (2014:e46) points out that STMMs have a history of "simply assuming the care provided is safe and has minimal risks." And perhaps this turns out to be true; perhaps care provision was safe and not risky. But, as Sykes and Orlando both contend, there is always a possibility that clinical work at STMMs is not beneficial to the populations they serve. It is hard to imagine a domain of professional practice, particularly one related to medicine, where such a lack of accountability and information would be considered either tolerable or ethical, let alone be embraced by medical professionals. But in a place where volunteers imagine that there is no doctor (whether or not this is so), good enough becomes good enough. And as we have seen in this chapter, in a place where there is no feedback about outcomes and no real engagement with place, confidence in one's own professional abilities allows good enough to become good.

# Conclusion

*Affect and Critical Global Health Research That Matters*

Attention to our intimate connections with our own actions reveals affect as a generative force in contemporary global health. In this conclusion, I first review how affect generally and visceral ethics specifically drive DIY global health. Affect frequently stands in when contextual knowledge is lacking, bolstering volunteers' confidence in their belief that global health work is righteous work. I then explore why we should be apprehensive about assuming that STMMs contribute positively to volunteers' ethical lives. Ultimately my work on affect has opened up new possibilities for critical scholars to communicate about global health in ways that matter to publics that are considering their own global health experience.

## Affect as a Generative Force in Global Health

I began my interview with Luke, a doctor who had volunteered at numerous STMMs in Guatemala over several years, by asking him to tell me about his mission work and how he got involved. The interview became dramatic quickly, as he recounted several incredible stories, including the following, which concerned "ma[king] a huge difference in two kids' lives":

> LUKE: We were in this town in northern Guatemala and learning, both
> from the people and just from reading, these people had had—what's
> the Latin word?—they had had the shit kicked out of 'em for forty
> years by the government. The Mayans were just absolutely deci-
> mated. . . . We were there for two weeks, that first time. Somehow,
> we were contacted by a Canadian nurse. . . . He found out we were
> in town and approached the leader of our group and said, "Can we

borrow your doctor for two days? There's a village north of here, and we want to screen the kids." We got volunteered. We get in the bus, just the nurse and a few doctors, I think, one or two other people, and we set up basically a miniclinic in a schoolroom in this village. This village had been the epicenter of the abuse and the massacres of the Mayans, of the Indians. . . . We set up, and we saw 165 kids over two days. It was the first time most of 'em had ever seen a doctor in their lives. They were from five to eleven years old. Anyway, [two] of us picked up . . . child[ren] with some peculiar cardiac murmurs. . . . Because the Canadian guy was a nurse, we said, "Listen. We'd like these two kids to be seen in Guatemala City. Something's going on." [Later] we got feedback on them. Both those kids made it to Guatemala City, and both ended up having open-heart surgery to correct some pretty bad problems that would've ended their lives early.

I can't tell you—I can't tell you how—I get emotional about it. When I got the feedback six months later that these kids had had surgery, . . . [that made] all five years of our trips down there . . . worthwhile. Understand that, for these kids to get to Guatemala City, it meant that one of their parents had to stay in the village to take care of the other kids and the goats and the chickens. Another parent got on a bus for about a ten-hour trip to Guatemala City. Those kids were evaluated within a month and a half of our visit. Then, within six months, both had open-heart surgery, when some of those American surgical teams came down. For those people— and I may be overdramatizing it—but for those people to submit, to go to all that trouble, based on our word, and then to submit to having their child's chest opened by a foreign doctor, I can only imagine what a cultural gulf that was for them. Again, I'm over-dramatizing, perhaps, but . . . for them to have your chest opened and exploring your heart goes back to Aztec times, when that was a sacrificial thing. I don't want to overdramatize it. I just thought the cultural gulf had to be huge.

NICOLE: Right. The trust that had to exist somewhere in that chain is pretty impressive.

LUKE: It was. It's been six years, Nicole, and I can't tell you. I've talked about it before, but right now I'm pretty emotional, thinking about it. That made all the effort and all the hundreds of people that we saw, that made it worthwhile and convinced me that what we were doing was not just dallying in Third World misery. It made a huge difference in two kids' lives.

I do not begrudge Luke his deep feelings of accomplishment for having positively changed the lives of two children forever. I share his sense of awe reflecting on the trust it took for each of these families to hear news about their children from a random stranger and to act on that information. I find it all the more remarkable because heart surgery is particularly invasive and scary, and these families probably faced numerous barriers in accessing care (Flood et al., 2018). Nonetheless, I would like to reflect on the fact that Luke draws conclusions about five years of work from a couple of successes. From a professional lens, a clinician judging the merits of the care they provide on the basis of merely two (successful) cases would be unacceptable in their home country, so why would one do so abroad?

Luke's newfound conviction about his global health work stemming from feelings related to these two cases reminds me of my own jornada-related myopia. I still clearly remember Antonia and how the removal of the debilitating cyst from her abdomen caused my feelings of awe and accomplishment. Indeed, her case has stood out for me as an overwhelming success. Just as Luke's evaluation of the worth of his action is mute regarding the other cases he intervened in, until I started to cross-examine my own feelings about my actions at jornadas, I did not remember the vast majority of the cases that I had seen, nor did I think about what happened to Antonia after she left the jornada. Most of the cases, including hers, closed for me after her successful surgery. Here we can clearly see visceral ethics at play. Our feelings of success can provide the gut security that our global health action is good, resulting in a lack of curiosity regarding the actual impacts on people or their health.

Frank, a doctor I met at a conference, told me a story that further encapsulates the importance of affect in shaping contemporary global health. Frank had been involved in a medical mission that began as a small group of physician colleagues traveling to the same area every year. They eventually formed a full-fledged NGO to fund themselves, and Frank served on the board of directors. I was surprised when Frank told me that he quit the board due to a disagreement and no longer volunteered with the organization. The disagreement surrounded a proposal to build a permanent clinic that volunteers could work out of during their missions. Frank was not opposed to a clinic per se. Yet he felt that before making a decision, the board needed an evaluation of how the clinic might impact people's access to care. Indeed, a hospital, which had not existed when Frank first started going on this mission, had been built nearby in ensuing years. He was concerned that building a new clinic, staffed with constant waves of foreign volunteers, might endanger the economic viability of the permanent hospital and undercut people's access to year-round, sustainable care. The other board members thought that an evaluation was unnecessary as they were positive that building a clinic was a good thing to do. Ultimately, the board executed their decision to build the clinic without any evaluation of the impact on access to care for people living in the area, and Frank quit.

Frank's reflection demonstrates how feelings of people working in the domain can become constitutive of global health. As we have seen, contemporary global health increasingly includes new players engaged in DIY global health work; why and how they contribute to global health becomes tied to their own views of doing good in the world (see also Schnable, 2021). Frank's example demonstrates how feelings of the board of directors about the goodness of the work that they were doing drove the building of a new clinic and resulted in a plethora of new global health volunteer opportunities. In the DIY domain, the intent to do good works can be tightly bound to deep feelings about the goodness of the work. Indeed, these feelings are sufficient to justify new projects and interventions. Affect becomes a creative force shaping global health.

I opened this conclusion with Luke's and Frank's stories because they summarize and support key points that I have made in this book. Affective experiences can be more critical to galvanizing DIY global health than any empirical data or outcomes. STMMs are not the result of formal assessments of unmet need, nor are their outputs typically tracked to see clinical results or epidemiological analyses. Medical missions in Sololá are more driven by volunteers' ideas of a place that is poor, Indigenous, and lacking care than by empirical realities and are driven also by their ideas that global health action can, at the very least, make one life better. This potential of doing good converts STMMs from just a professional opportunity to an opportunity for volunteers to build their ethical lives. Responding to privilege in their own lives (and in the lives of their children) by helping people with fewer opportunities is a central attraction of STMMs. Once at a medical mission, the patina of helping others is ever present and palpable for volunteers. With an absence of contextual information, volunteers rely on their own professional competence, reinforced by their ideas of place, to make sense of events. With the absence of information needed to assess the morality of their actions, volunteers rely on visceral ethics to judge the good they do. Visceral ethics can make things feel right, regardless of whether volunteers' judgments are connected to anything real.

## STMMs and Moral Vulnerability of Volunteers: Unintended Harms and Lack of Accountability

We should be deeply concerned about how affect might be circumventing attention to negative impacts of DIY global health. I illustrate this point by considering three different levels at which STMMs can cause harm. At the personal level, clinicians, who are trying to build their ethical lives, may cause unintended harm to their patients at STMMs, harms that they may be unable to recognize and redress. At the population level, STMMs may have further negative impacts on already-stressed health systems. STMMs also contribute to problematic arrangements in the global health domain itself, arrangements that contravene what we know will be best for health equity. Each of these issues is addressed in turn in this section.

As seen in Luke's story and in Claudia's story shared in chapter 5, clinicians involved in STMMs tend to evaluate the rightness of their actions at STMMs through the lens of what they accomplished in the clinic. In this calculus, good doctoring at a jornada is worthy, good action. The physician-anthropologist Anita Chary and physician David Flood (2021) complicate such a truncated analysis of whether a clinician's work is good work and not harmful to patients. They reflect on their own problematic experiences in the US of prescribing opioids, drugs that are currently fueling a public health crisis. Opioids provide excellent pain relief, but as Chary and Flood argue, they can also prompt "cascade iatrogenesis," or progressively more harmful medical decisions for patients. While standards of care may support prescribing opioids, Chary and Flood explore the distress they feel as physicians when their own actions contribute to further harms to patients. Rather than placing our focus on individual clinical decision-making, Chary and Flood insist that physicians' ability to make decisions consonant with their own moral dispositions must be analyzed with reference to the bureaucracies and structures in which they work. More specifically, they draw on the Austrian philosopher Ivan Illich (1975) to highlight the roles of these structures in naturalizing risks that harm patients.

To adapt Chary and Flood's point, a volunteer's evaluation of their own clinical proficiency at an STMM is inadequate to understand potential harm to patients; we need to consider how STMMs structure clinical work and naturalize risk for patients. As a short-term model, STMMs build in numerous risks. An oft-commented concern voiced by Guatemalan and North American interviewees as well as in literatures on the ethics of STMMs concerns the lack of continuity of care or adequate follow-up endemic to the short-term model (Nouvet, Chan, & Schwartz, 2018; Zientek & Bonnell, 2020). Building a model of practice around leaving any patient behind, particularly a surgical one, compromises quality care. Even if a jornada goes back to the same place, it does not typically reach out to prior patients for follow-up. Moreover, there is no guarantee that the clinician whom a patient originally saw would be present. Patients who are left behind by an STMM need better self-care and monitoring plans than do patients who have continued access to care locally. But producing tangible, written plans would be challenging for volunteers given the language differences that typify the short-term model.[1] Furthermore, it takes time to produce an adequate plan (e.g., one that accurately reflects health literacy) and to explain it, time that would significantly cut the number of patients a clinician could see.[2] But the lack of plans means that patients are more at risk for not taking their drugs correctly, not caring for themselves postsurgery, and missing early signs of complications. If patients cannot count on follow-up and do not have good care and monitoring plans, they need excellent records of diagnosis and treatment to seek care from local providers. But again, this does not typically happen. Patients do not leave jornadas with preoperative and diagnostic labs that they could give to local providers. Volunteers frequently do not have skills needed to produce records in the language of the host country. Also, STMMs are frequently barebones operations. They do not have time or money to send patients out for diagnostic procedures or the ability to do them on-site. Patients at jornadas I accompanied did not receive medical records. Indeed, I found that post-op surgical patients at STMMs in Sololá could typically not describe their clinical diagnosis or the surgery they received.[3] Sparse equipment at STMMs can limit the ability of the clinical team to handle medical emergencies as well as they could be handled in a public hospital. These are only a handful of ethical issues inherent in the ways STMMs are structured, creating extra risk to patients and thus leading to increased likelihood of harms.[4]

The extra risks to patients stemming from how STMMs are structured are all the more concerning given the difficulties of detecting or recognizing unintended harms. The physician David Addiss and the public health scholar Joseph Amon (2019) identify four barriers impeding professionals' ability to recognize unintended harms in the global health domain. Three of these barriers are prominent in STMMs: inadequate surveillance, power imbalances, and self-image.[5] I have argued that during DIY global health action, our own feelings in the moment that our work is good substitute for the short-, mid-, and long-term monitoring of patient outcomes characteristic of professional clinical practice in brick-and-mortar clinical spaces nearly anywhere in the world. Addiss and Amon further explain how the power dynamics inherent to global health interventions can create a barrier to recognizing harm. Much global health work, STMMs included, are characterized by well-off people traveling to new places to assist those who are less well off. Yet Addiss and Amon (2019:24) suggest, "it may be difficult for persons who occupy positions of power and wealth to recognize the impact of unintended harm when it occurs in someone who is already marginalized, geographically distant." Finally, recognizing unintended harms can conflict with one's ideas about oneself. Many people are prompted to global health action by the value of solidarity with others as well as the idea that they are doing good work. This very self-image "creates powerful internal incentives for discounting evidence that one's actions have had unintended adverse consequences" (Addiss & Amon, 2019:24).

Furthermore, patients who are unintentionally harmed are more typically vulnerable than they would be otherwise because of the structural issues with STMMs. Most STMMs are quasi-legal or illegal in host countries, a fact frequently ignored by volunteers and organizers. Of primary concern is that licensed North American clinicians are not licensed to practice in the foreign countries where STMMs occur. Because they are not licensed in those locations, they are not regulated or insured. Moreover, they typically follow their own standards of care rather than those in the host country. In addition, Virginia Rowthorn et al. (2019) point out that STMMs also frequently run afoul of host-country drug laws, such as importing drugs illegally or dispensing expired drugs. This can create many complications for patients.[6] The anthropologist Mary Catherine Driese (2022) finds that in Guatemala, where malpractice laws are weak and taking legal action for medical harm is complicated, patients who are harmed at a jornada frequently lack adequate documentation to hold an STMM accountable. Even in countries with better malpractice protection than Guatemala, culpable volunteers are probably not in the country or insured, making redressing harm difficult. Likewise, the STMMs and NGOs that volunteers are affiliated with are frequently not legal entities in host countries but in HICs, where they can get charitable status and tax benefits. This leaves patients little protection or recourse.

In sum, at the clinical level, STMMs are quite concerning. Ample professional clinical skill is not sufficient to guarantee an absence of harms.[7] Indeed, extra risks to patients are built into the structures of STMMs. Furthermore, there are important barriers to recognizing or acknowledging unintended harms stemming from STMMs. Were harms to be perpetrated and recognized in STMM work, there are no good protocols concerning how individual clinicians or STMMs themselves could be held accountable or redress those harms.[8]

While clinical care may create unintended harm for patients, STMMs can also have harmful impacts on the care available to patients outside of the jornada. As travel to rural and remote areas lacking care is difficult for volunteers, jornadas typically take place in areas (like Sololá) where patients already have access to public and private care (Driese, 2022). In short, STMMs often duplicate available existing clinical services, even though volunteers may be unaware that this is the case. Another issue that came up in conversations with Guatemalan doctors was STMMs undercutting the livelihoods of local, private health care providers.[9]

Working in the public sector paid little, and doctors earned far more in their private clinics; however, there was a limited number of patients who could pay. For this reason, many doctors made ends meet by working part-time in the public system and part-time in their own private clinic. As we have seen, people from many socioeconomic backgrounds, including both Indigenous and Ladino people who could afford private care, sought attention at jornadas. Reducing demand for private care by treating patients at a jornada could negatively impact physicians and thus have negative knock-on effects on care provided in the public sector, including predatory behavior (e.g., physicians increasing pressure on patients in the public hospital to see them in their private practices), decreased quality of care (as physicians downgrade the quality of care they provide in the public sector to make adequate care only available for a fee), and increased absenteeism (as physicians supplement their income with paid work during hours when they are supposed to be serving the public) (Ferrinho et al., 2004).

Furthermore, STMMs create an optic for care that is impractical and unsustainable, which may cause further harms by undercutting citizens' faith in the Guatemalan health system. In comparison to the public system, STMMs have no shortages or stock-outs as volunteers bring all supplies that they think they need. Volunteers offer free care and free medications. STMMs do not require any of the cumbersome and expensive labs and tests required for treatment by Guatemalan health care providers. A patient can move from triage to surgery quickly, sometimes in less than a day. But these characteristics are created by volunteers operating in ways that they would not and could not at home. For example, if you need elective surgery in Canada, there tend to be long wait times; in the US, health care is not affordable, making it inaccessible to many people. Nevertheless, patients at jornadas do not necessarily know or understand that corners are cut or that the care offered does not necessarily mirror the conditions of health systems in North America. Rather as many patients assume that foreign professionals from HICs are better trained (Citrin, 2010; Green et al., 2009; Mantey et al., 2021; Nouvet, Chan, & Schwartz, 2018), they may perceive the convenience of a well-working jornada as what really good health care looks like, in spite of the reality that the care may not meet minimum standards in Guatemala, let alone in the home countries of the STMM clinicians (Wendland, 2012).

The STMM model relies on many aspects of formal global health interventions that have been called out for undercutting LMIC health systems (Pfeiffer & Nichter, 2008; Prince & Otieno, 2014; Storeng, 2014). For example, STMMs create better-funded structures in parallel to public health systems, rather than in support of public systems. STMM care is typically focused on specific issues (which can be addressed over the course of a week or two) rather than offering or strengthening comprehensive primary care. Examining surgical missions from the position of someone from a LMIC, the surgeon Alberto Ferreres (2022) critiques the ethics of the short-term model of care. He reminds us that while there may be a shortage of surgeons in LMICs, patients in LMICs have a fundamental right to a sustainable and reliable health care system that can provide needed surgical care. Stopgap measures, like surgical missions, violate a number of patients' rights while doing nothing to strengthen their access to sustainable care. Ferreres's rejection of the idea that STMMs can function ethically is reminiscent of important work by the anthropologist Ramah McKay (2017). McKay refers to "medicine in the meantime," describing how people involved in the global health domain rationalize projects and processes that admittedly circumvent practices necessary to promote the health systems within the countries in which they work.[10] A classic example of this comes from Matthew C. Davis et al. (2014), who analyze the cost-effectiveness of flying foreign surgeons to Guatemala to address the nation's neurosurgical needs. While it might be cost-effective from a budgetary standpoint, this is precisely the sort of voluntary, charity-based solution that Ferreres identifies as undercutting Guatemalans' basic rights to safe, sustainable (and, I would argue, dignified) care. Both McKay and Ferreres emphasize that global health projects can either sustain inequitable practices undermining health systems or enact transformational practices that would bolster those systems—there is no middle ground "in the meantime" where makeshift, inequitable global health work is helpful.

Scholars, practitioners, and students have been pushing to decolonize global health and have highlighted how colonial ways of thinking inspire global health action and perpetuate inequities (Abimbola & Pai, 2020; Gautier et al., 2022; Khan et al., 2021; Kwete et al., 2022; Mogaka, Stewart, & Bukusi, 2021). Lara Gautier et al. (2022:184) describe colonial ways of thinking as "a set of internalized ideas, values, attitudes, perceptions, and beliefs rooted in colonial logic, that grounds systems of hierarchies, knowledge and culture, in this particular case, between the West and its former colonies in modern history."[11] Volunteers have learned and practice medicine in a system that is marked by colonialism (Cohen-Fournier, Brass, & Kirmayer, 2021; Smith-Morris et al., 2021; Turpel-Lafond & Johnson, 2021) and can bring colonial ways of thinking to Guatemalan clinical encounters.

Even though volunteers are attracted to global health action to express solidarity and promote health equity, DIY global health (including STMMs) remains rooted in a basic colonial logic—namely, that people from North America need to take care of people in poor countries as they are unable to take care of themselves (a.k.a. the White man's burden; Bandyopadhyay, 2019). This results in troubling colonial power inequities between volunteers and patients, which enables volunteers to define both the problems and the solutions.[12] While negative (racial) stereotyping is hopefully rare in STMMs, inequities between volunteers and patients can translate into less-than-safe care, particularly for Indigenous peoples. In the case of medical missions, where patients are not paying for care and volunteers are not being paid for their service, some patients may be even more reluctant to "question" their care provider (Roche et al., 2018). At the same time, these power inequities undercut provider accountability (Addis and Amon, 2019) and make it more difficult for patients to receive care in the way that they prefer or need (Driese, 2022).

The physician and health system researcher Seye Abimbola and the physician and epidemiologist Madhukar Pai (2020) help us identify the difference between global health predicated on colonial visions and solidarity. They describe an imagined world where global health has been decolonized and "recognises that you cannot truly help or support people, be their allies and enablers, without seeing the world through their eyes and seeing yourself as they see you" (Abimbola & Pai, 2020:1628). You must get to know someone and share experiences and conversations to be able to "see . . . through their eyes" and to be able to "see . . . yourself as they see you" (Abimbola & Pai, 2020:1628). Solidarity is necessarily built through relationships and reflection. But DIY global health is designed to be ephemeral, lacking the continuity required to develop meaningful relationships and exchanges between "yourself" and "them" that could lead to solidarity. Decolonizing global health depends on transformations that make the thoughts, ideas, experiences, and perspectives of recipients of global health programming as important to structuring global health as those of people in HICs. Clearly, when considered from these sorts of standards, DIY global health is a regressive practice, and its actual contribution to volunteers' ethical lives needs to be more closely interrogated.

## Reframing Critical Global Health Scholarship: Meeting People "Where They Are"

As I have argued in this book, there is a mismatch between the way critical scholars of global health tend to approach the global health domain and the way many people doing applied work within that domain view it. My colleagues and I have focused largely on systems and relations underwriting global health and have tried to address inequities through critique. Our work reveals the lack of justice in contemporary practice and disjunctures between what global health seeks to do and what is actually occurring (Benton, 2015; Berry, 2010; Biruk, 2018; Fan, 2021; Kalofonos, 2021; McKay, 2017; Nguyen, 2010). But what if individuals engaging in global health action work in a space that is focused on (clinical) competence alone? What if they understand their activities on the basis of strong feelings stemming from one moment or selective cases of success? In this case, scholarly critiques of historical, political, and social complexities contributing to global health failures fall flat. Two totally different understandings and conversations are occurring, each separate from the other.

I have observed this disconnect firsthand during this research. The jornada organizers and volunteers with whom I spoke were skeptical, as well as curious, intelligent, and engaged—ideal qualities for interlocutors.[13] Many volunteers prepared for a jornada by reading everything they could get their hands on about history and society in Guatemala; indeed, volunteers asked me for my research papers and/or my first book, which they heartily devoured. But they did not see my context-rich approach to Sololá as telling a cautionary tale that could fundamentally inform their own global health work. Rather, my research fell into a toolkit they used to more closely tailor jornadas to locale. This was frustrating for me, because, as Frank pointed out earlier, the idea of doing it better is an insufficiently skeptical goal, as it truncates necessary questions, such as, "Should we be doing it at all?"

In the classroom, I regularly (and successfully) navigate this gap between my critical approach to global health and students who want to do something good in the world. Actually, I look forward to navigating this gap. In the classroom, I want people to learn. In fact, I view my job as providing students with learning opportunities. Respect is crucial to creating environments where students learn; that respect would be undermined if I viewed my job as trying to change their minds or labeling their values as right or wrong. When students express ideas about global health or come to me to consider global health placements, I do not give them an elevator speech about research on structural inequities in global health. Instead, I tend to ask questions that highlight important dynamics that they might not be thinking about. Indeed, this is a key strategy that my colleagues and I routinely use to make teaching relevant and is encapsulated by the phrase "meet students where they are."

If we want critical, anthropological research to matter to those who are doing applied global health, we need to take a page from our teaching, reconsidering our audiences and where they are. Because I assign critical global health scholarship in class, I am acutely aware that students need me to contextualize, bridge, and translate what is at stake in order for this scholarship to contribute significantly to their learning. Indeed, much of the global health scholarship that I enjoy and assign is primarily written for me—someone employed as a professor working in a university with expertise in the field.

My research on affective dimensions of global health has shown the importance of our intimate connections—that is, our own feelings about the actions we take—to the global health domain. This is where our audience is. Feelings have also frequently been overlooked as important in our critical scholarship. While pointing to empirical realities of place (e.g., lack of need for a new clinic or even harm done by building one) might not substantially influence how volunteers plan their global health engagements, prompting changes in their *own feelings* about global health action being a good idea could. (Professional) volunteers will not be drawn to global health experiences that they feel do not contribute positively to their own ethical lives. As Frank, Alexander, and other volunteers with whom I spoke demonstrated, such global health experiences lose their allure.

I see my work on visceral ethics as contributing to an accessible framing of critical global health that meets wider publics where they are. Visceral ethics highlights how affective dimensions stand in the way of global health volunteers becoming accountable for their actions. In Sololá, volunteers can practice medicine in ways that they would never be comfortable with in their home countries, blinded to everything except the immediate cases facing them, with little risk that they will be held accountable for the consequences of their actions—neither in Guatemala nor at their "real" jobs at home.[14] This lack of accountability becomes possible when global health programming is imagined and executed outside of the formal systems that exist in the places where STMMs operate and, as Abimbola and Pai (2020) contend, without meaningful consultation and input from communities.[15]

Current movements toward equity worldwide have paved the way for anthropological insight into global health to matter to wider publics. In North America, where many budding global health volunteers and I live, our current social milieu is characterized by crucial social movements that have brought *systemic* inequities into daily public conversations.[16] For instance, in the United States, amplified by the murder of George Floyd, the Black Lives Matter movement and the *New York Times'* "1619 Project" have highlighted for a wider public the realities of systemic racial inequality. The 2015 report of the Truth and Reconciliation Commission in Canada has provided the public with unprecedented access to First Nations people's accounts of physical, psychological, and systemic violence suffered at residential schools, reinforced by the recent discovery of children's graves on former residential school grounds. Canada is now rife with information on how ongoing settler violence over stolen Indigenous lands and resources results in wider anti-Indigenous racism both at the community level and within justice and health systems nationwide. As public interest in understanding these wider systemic inequities has grown, authors have written several outstanding, bestselling books that have captured wider imaginations in a way that excellent earlier scholarship did not (Kendi, 2019; King, 2017; Oluo, 2019; Simpson, 2020). These books have opened conversations about how privilege works to create unearned advantages for some at the expense of others and have inspired many of us in North America to reflect more deeply on how our own privilege contributes to harm. Furthermore, the role of privileged people's affect in upholding systems of inequity has also been a major part of these conversations (Anderson, 2016; Morrison, 2017).

My arguments about how visceral ethics works in relation to global health bridges into these public conversations. My privilege protects my comfort. Similarly, visceral ethics functions like a balm that can soothe volunteers' doubts about the moral nature of their action. In a moment that stresses how people need to unlearn and embrace feeling unsettled, that visceral ethics (re)creates comfort should serve as a red flag. This red flag signals that volunteers need to scrutinize long-standing presumptions about what doing good work as a clinician abroad looks like as well as consider more deeply unintentional harms that can stem from a lack of accountability to populations that are already disenfranchised. Undoubtedly, this was one of the Nigerian-American novelist Teju Cole's (2012) central messages in calling out the "White Saviour Industrial Complex." And this is a responsibility that, at minimum, should be a central concern to people who might want to engage in global health work.

Meeting publics interested in DIY global health where they are means starting from the point that volunteers want to take action that helps them build their own ethical lives. We can encourage a more fulsome evaluation of the relevance of STMMs to volunteers' ethical lives by focusing on volunteers' own moral vulnerability. For reasons discussed earlier, medical missions may make volunteers morally vulnerable—that is, place them in situations in which they may inadvertently perpetrate unintended harms on people who are less privileged than themselves, while simultaneously protecting volunteers from any consequences. Yet volunteers typically do not think about the risks that STMMs create for patients or how STMMs produce harms beyond immediate clinical care. This means that volunteers are not consciously considering the difference between STMMs that function in agreement with their own moral beliefs and STMMs that create harms that exceed a volunteer's own threshold for good work.

Advocating for meeting volunteers at their own moral vulnerability is qualitatively different from current go-to approaches, like the Brocher Declaration (Prasad et al., 2022), aiming to secure good works in the DIY domain.[17] The Brocher Declaration emphasizes key principles that organizations should meet for ethical, sustainable, and equitable short-term global health experiences like STMMs. I agree with the importance of the key principles outlined, and they certainly can be used by volunteers as a guideline regarding which types of STMMs they should or should not align themselves with. But like critical scholarship in global health, this sort of approach needs to be bridged to be useful. For instance, the Brocher Declaration is not presented in a form that prompts a volunteer to undertake the due diligence necessary to figure out which STMMs uphold a volunteer's own moral beliefs and which STMMs create the potential for harms that go beyond a volunteer's comfort level.[18]

What sorts of questions could prompt a more thorough consideration of dynamics that determine the ethical value of a STMM to a volunteer? First, we need an approach that highlights the necessity for a thorough due diligence as the responsibility of volunteers (not organizers or friends or webpages or other rhetorics that volunteers might be tempted to rely on as a proxy for what is going on). My research has demonstrated how volunteers can fail to investigate important ethical actions of STMMs before participating (e.g., Do they screen at the door for poor, Indigenous patients, or are they arranging activities to build Indigenous self-determination?). Furthermore, Driese (2022) recounts an important example of an STMM organizer who hired an on-the-ground staff member in Guatemala and just assumed that the staff member was following through on what needed to be done, including securing the legal right for North American volunteer clinicians to practice in Guatemala. In her example, we see that when asked, an organizer in good faith reported that the STMM had met local legal requirements, when in fact this was not the case. As Teresa so poignantly phrased it, in the world of medical missions, "you be sure." Given that many organizations and persons rely on visceral ethics that short-circuit a fulsome investigation of and reflection on action, due diligence in the DIY domain falls to the volunteer. Second, we need an approach that emphasizes individual variability in the importance of aspects of STMMs that connect to ethics. By highlighting key principles, the Brocher Declaration keeps our attention focused on unified agreement. This approach papers over sources of moral vulnerability for individual volunteers, a focus that is important for helping volunteers navigate which DIY opportunities are actually consonant with the type of action they want to undertake.

We now turn to examples of how to build on insights from both critical scholarship and key principle approaches, to prompt volunteers' due diligence and emphasize individual moral vulnerability. For example, providing care to vulnerable populations that do not normally have access is a major reason that clinicians see STMMs as contributing to their ethical lives.[19] Nevertheless, most STMMs just assume that they are accomplishing this.[20] Questions that might prompt a volunteer toward a more thorough evaluation of whether populations without access are being reached include the following:

- Most STMMs do not do thorough epidemiologic analyses or review available care resources before choosing a place to go. How do you know you will serve people who do not have access to care? Geographically, what parts of the host country for the STMM experience the most health inequities? What sorts of health care is lacking in the STMM area? What information have you found that suggests the STMM will be providing needed health resources that do not already exist?
- Affordability is one necessary but not sufficient condition to make care accessible to disenfranchised populations. What typical barriers affect disenfranchised populations in the country and area of the STMM? What actions is the STMM taking to address these barriers and make care accessible for disenfranchised populations? How does it know that these actions help?

Another area that figures prominently in clinicians' ethical lives is following best professional practices. Examples of questions that dig deeper into this area and emphasize moral lines that a volunteer might not want to cross include the following:

- Allowing local communities to have a say in their own health care is important. What specific processes does this STMMs set in place to ensure that local communities can provide critical feedback and shape future STMMs?

How has the jornada worked locally to ensure that the local community's ideas and perspectives are reflected in the STMM? Can you provide an example of how this engagement has changed or adapted the provision of care in the STMM? What are areas that organizers and the community are still concerned about? How do you feel about those concerns?

- What is the legality of the STMM? Have you investigated current bans or restrictions on STMMs in the host country? If you are going to be practicing legally, who is taking responsibility for you and why? Whose responsibility is it to show you the official permission before you practice? Would you be willing to take legal responsibility for a local doctor coming to your practice or hospital next week and seeing patients on their own? If not, what do you think is different about the dynamic when you travel to a different country?

- If you are practicing illegally, what do you think would be the risks if a doctor from the host country came to your town and practiced without license or insurance? What risks does you practicing illegally at an STMM create for patients, for local health care providers, or for local clinics and hospitals? What steps are you taking to mitigate negative impacts of those risks on patients?

- Will you be importing drugs in your luggage as part of the STMM? Will any of these drugs be expired? Are they all available in the host country? What is the legality of importing the drugs you will bring into the host country? How would you feel about bringing and dispensing drugs that are illegal in the host country?

A third area of import to clinicians' ethical lives is doing no harm. Yet, as discussed, STMMs are frequently structured in ways that create harms for patients, and volunteers assume that because organizers and other volunteers think the STMM is doing good, this must be true. Examples of questions that draw out this dynamic include the following:

- Practicing in a different context can create different risks for patients. What have you learned about how practicing at the STMM will create risks? What risks will patients at the STMM face that are not typical for those you see in your own clinic? What is your comfort level with additional risks? Why? Can you think of a way that patients in the host country could get care without these additional risks? How could you facilitate that care?

- Additional risks make leaving good self-care and monitoring plans for patients as well as records of the care that patients received at STMMs critically important. Do patients at the STMM have literacy or language needs that are not typical of patients in your clinic at home? If so, describe these needs. Detail your plan for meeting patients' needs for useful plans. How will you know if it is working or not? What sorts of information will host-country health care workers need to follow up with a patient you treat? How do you know?

- What information and feedback do you depend on in your own practice to ensure the quality of care that you offer? What information and feedback will you depend on at the STMM? If it differs from what you have access to at home, do you consider it adequate? Why or why not?

- What will happen to a patient who suffers unintentional harm under your care? How will you find out about the harm? What is your plan to redress any harm you create? What happens if you have already returned home when you learn that you unintentionally harmed a patient?

These questions provide a few examples of how this research on affective dimensions of global health can be used to strategize meeting potential global health volunteers at their desire to do good in the world. Combined with knowledge about visceral ethics, these sorts of questions can dampen the affective allure of DIY global health work and prompt volunteers to consider the information that they actually need to evaluate the likelihood that STMMs contribute to a life they want to lead.

Asking questions such as "How do you know?" also moves volunteers away from relying on reputations of STMMs to ensure due diligence. Volunteers and organizers frequently assume that they are going to a place where care is needed, that permissions have been obtained, that someone is ensuring that patients in need are the ones being seen, that plans for follow-up care have been handled, and that patients are better off than they were before the STMM.[21] Making such assumptions is the first step in doing unintentional harm. After decades of working in Guatemala, Teresa, the physician whose story I related in chapter 4, learned a critical lesson for STMM volunteers. The safety of patients depends on volunteers not farming out responsibility for gathering information but rather on doing that work themselves.

## The Importance of Addressing Affect in Global Health

Ethnographers of global health have tended to neglect its affective dimensions. This neglect is not inconsequential and is at the center of a major disconnect with publics that we want to engage. Our context-rich critiques of global health structures are, of course, valuable. However, if our aim is for anthropology to "matter," we must be sensitive to our audiences—not just fellow academics but rather the "doers" in the global health domain. We need to fundamentally reorient how we talk about problematic ethics and systemic inequities in global health. We need to write and speak in a way that helps our audiences make connections between their actions and the problematic ways that those actions could cause harm to people on the ground. Ignoring affect rather than understanding affect as integral and constitutive of global health is done not only at our peril but at the peril of the very equity-deserving communities we care about. By writing about visceral ethics, I hope I have convinced you that we need to take seriously the intentions of people who engage in global health action and meet them where they are.[22]

# ACKNOWLEDGMENTS

I would have never been able to write this book were it not for the generosity and support of many different people and organizations. I have been fortunate to receive substantial funding and support for my research in Guatemala over the past two decades. The impetus for this project and many of the foundational experiences, relationships, and understandings occurred during my dissertation fieldwork, and my field notes just keep on giving. I would like to thank the University of Michigan and all of its various departments and institutes that were central to supporting my education and my research leading me to a fruitful career as an anthropologist. I would also like to thank USED Fulbright-Hays and Wenner-Gren for their financial support of my early work. The Social Science and Humanities Research Council of Canada provided funding for more recent fieldwork and contributed greatly to this project.

For the past fifteen years, I have had the pleasure of teaching at Simon Fraser University and the Faculty of Health Sciences. This position has provided me with the time, space, and resources to do work that I love. I want to thank my wonderful colleagues who allow me to plop down in their offices to chat and whose care and attention always enrich the perspectives I can bring to my work. Specifically, I appreciate the open doors of my hall buddies, Angela Kaida, Jeremy Snyder, and Scott Venners, as well as Meghan Winters and her ready walking shoes. Maya Gislason's great idea of reserving room 11808 on Friday mornings to parallel write was essential to helping me establish a writing routine needed to actually complete a draft of this book.

I wrote this book over the three years that I served as associate dean in my faculty. In some ways, taking on an onerous administrative role that could have sucked up all my time made me more aggressive about protecting time to write. I would not have been able to routinely carve out time for my work if not for the amazing staff in the Faculty of Health

Sciences who supported the associate dean's work, including Rehana Bacchus, Robyn Bailey, Brad Mladenovic, Lucania Rad, and Kellie Smith.

I would also like to thank the Xʷməθkʷəy̓əm (Musquem), Sḵwx̱wú7mesh Úxwumixw (Squamish), səlilwətaɬ (Tsleil-Waututh), and kʷikʷəƛ̓əm (Kwikwetlem) peoples on whose unceded lands I live and wrote this book. I am particularly indebted for the millennia of steward-ship for the forests on Burnaby Mountain. Starting every day by walking these forests has given me the physical strengthen, mental clarity, and sense of peace needed to write.

Even though this is a book predominantly about North Americans, I relied on many friends and colleagues in Guatemala to do my research. None of this would have been possible without the kindness and help of those who live in Santa Cruz. The community of NGO- and STMM-affiliated friends and acquaintances in Panajachel were incredibly gen-erous with their time and connections. I also thank my Guatemalan colleagues for continuing to be supportive of my research. More specifi-cally, I would like to thank Dr. Georgina Monzón for allowing access to clinicians, hospital reports, and patients at San Juan de Dios Hospital in Sololá and Dr. Constantino Isaac Sánchez Montoya for facilitating access to interviewees who helped clarify important elements of this project. I am always grateful to Mayron Martinez and his support of research in the VIIth Health District. All of this detailed work helped me under-stand what I was studying and experiencing.

Because my research has always been so closely tied to Sololá, I have never had to do cold-calling before. I was nervous about tracking down strangers on the internet. What would they say when I asked to interview them or invited them to lunch? How would they understand my interest in joining their reunions or accompanying them to Guatemala? I was prepared to be rejected and ignored and even wrote a quick speech on "What is an anthropologist?" But this turned out to be unnecessary. I was astounded by the openness and generosity of people who shared their time, experience, bathrooms, and bunk rooms with me. I especially want to thank the organizations that found a place for me in their jornadas. I would never have been able to write this book without those experiences.

I am fortunate to have the support of many close colleagues who make my work far better. Michael Hathaway invited me to an all-day retreat to think about our second books and offered the insight that my second book did not have to be a rewrite of my first. This was psychologically transformational news that freed me to rip up the first several chapters I had produced early on (which were essentially just my first book, slightly rewritten). Michael has been a tireless consultant, always ready to jump into the middle of a chapter or issue and help me get unstuck. His encouragement to communicate with wider audiences is invaluable. I also want to thank Jessaca Leinaweaver for always being there. Her support and wisdom is priceless. I appreciate the critical and insightful feedback she provided on my very drafty first full draft. Page by page, it helped me rewrite, and I hope that I have been able to correct many of the issues that she identified. Rob Lorway was also generous enough to take time out during the first months of the pandemic to read my fledging manuscript. Thank you, Rob, for telling me things that I needed to hear. Jessaca and Michael were incredibly helpful when it came time to write a prospectus and reach out to presses. Even though I have been an academic for decades, there is still so much I do not know about publishing, particularly books. Thank you, Marcia Inhorn, for your sage advice and quick replies that enable me to navigate the publishing world. Any errors in these pages are certainly my own and do not reflect the superb advice or feedback that I have received.

I want to thank Jennifer Hammer at NYU Press, who saw the potential for this book and reinspired my enthusiasm to work on it again. Two anonymous reviewers have provided excellent guidance that helped me rethink and clarify what I was doing and how I was communicating it. This book is stronger because of them. I would also like to thank the editorial board for their supportive feedback and direction in revision.

As the dedication indicates, there would be no book without the tireless support and encouragement that I have received from Noelle Sullivan. The past several years have been challenging, and she was willing to stick with me throughout. I continue to be amazed by the depth of her insight into my own work and the anthropology of global health in general. I have profited immensely from her knowledge of clinical global health travel, an area that was new to me with this project. I am thankful that she has been willing to spend two hours a week with me over the past three and half years. I would never have kept going without her encouragement. It was Noelle who nudged me to consider how to relate visceral ethics, an idea nestled in chapter 3, into the rest of my book, and that insight was crucial to bringing this project together. She is a kind and clear critic. I hope that my feedback is as helpful to her as hers is to me.

Finally, I want to thank my family. I am grateful to my parents, Susanne and JB, and my most recent parent, Cynthia. JB and Cynthia provided a necessary soft landing for the kids that made it so much easier for us to move to Guatemala. I also appreciate having a quiet, safe room in their house where I could go "sleep it off" after a jornada. Sebastian and Lucas have been incredibly patient moving schools and countries and losing their mom for chunks of time all in the name of research. My husband, Pablo, has provided me with support and encouragement needed to get this done. Thank you, Pablo, for being there for me through the ups and the downs.

# NOTES

## PROLOGUE

1  While I have settled on this terminology, there are many ways that other people refer to what I am calling "medical missions," including "health camps" and "health brigades." I delve into my choice of terminology and the difference between medical missions and religious missions in chapter 1.

2  Biruk (2018) does an excellent job of unpacking and critiquing this "soap-for-information transaction." While the dynamics of ethnographic fieldwork are a bit different from the global health projects Biruk examines, I agree with their point that anthropologists can remain complicit in contributing to the social worlds we write about. I should note that gifting soap was my own choice, made predominantly for superficial and instrumental reasons. As Biruk points out, soap has great transportability; it was manageable for me to carry on the long hikes necessary to reach interviewees' houses and did not jeopardize my safety (as carrying and giving out cash might have). Soap is packed with local meaning, as it plays a role in family exchange and can be associated with guests and visitors—who in the best of circumstances are invited to enjoy a new bar of soap when washing their hands. Nonetheless, Guatemala, like Malawi, has a colonial history where there is a fraught relationship between hygiene, disease, and race. As a non-Indigenous person, I cannot gift soap unmoored from those histories.

3  *Jornada* literally means "day of work" or, more figuratively, "work shift" in Spanish. In this area in Guatemala, however, it is the colloquial term used to describe short-term medical missions, where doctors arrive and work for a day or a few days. Kaqchikel speakers borrowed the term from Spanish when referring to medical missions.

4  While Indigenous men frequently wore Western-style clothing, Indigenous women from villages in Sololá frequently wore traditional clothing. In this area of Sololá, *huipiles*, traditional blouses, are generally made from hand-woven cloth embroidered with designs and colors pertaining to a geographic location. *Cortes* are traditional skirts worn by Indigenous women. Buying the standard black cloth that the *corte* was made out of had become more popular than hand-weaving it. Like the *huipil*, this cloth was then frequently embroidered by hand with designs and colors that again pertained to particular geographic locations. Women's clothing was relatively expensive because of the money and time needed to make it.

5 Green et al. (2009), who also based their research in Sololá, address perceptions
of Guatemalans toward medical missions. They find, among other things, that
Guatemalan health care professionals sense a lack of respect of mission doctors
toward the Guatemalan health system and themselves.

6 In this chapter, I am intentionally vague about what is entailed in global health. I
develop and specify what I mean by "global health" in chapter 1.

## INTRODUCTION

1 In chapter 1, I clarify my use of the term "contemporary global health." Scholarly
constructions of this domain have tended to remain tightly focused on formal
endeavors (e.g., bilateral assistance, international organization). As I argue in
chapter 1, informal, "do-it-yourself" activities, like jornadas, now also characterize
contemporary global health activities.

2 This is, of course, a different claim than saying that global health action is really
improving the world. The actual effects of global health work can only be determined empirically. Assessing the positive or negative impacts of global health
work is beyond the scope of this book. My focus remains on what people think
that they have done.

3 This is not to say that *everyone* who works in global health has the same goals and
motivations. Lasker (2016) finds that many young people setting out for volunteer
global health placements are motivated by a desire to build their own curriculum
vitae or skills. In the professional realm, Pfeiffer (2003), for example, documents
"aid cowboys" or "aid mercenaries" who pervade the field. These are career global
health professionals who are drawn by the "war stories" or "the money," not their
desire to help.

4 Dave's rendition of affect aligns closely with critical scholarship on affect theory
that also emphasizes affect as primordial or unconscious, a counterpoint to the
intentional rationality ascribed to semiotic theory (Navaro-Yashin, 2009; Newell, 2018; Skoggard & Waterston, 2015). Her work is theoretically inspirational
for me because she identifies how the primordialness or nascentness of affect
allows incommensurability with the real world and becomes a creative force.
This step is critically important in understanding how a volunteer's deep feeling
of having done something good in the world can be creative and trump the need
for an empirical evaluation of the actual effects of participating in an medical
mission.

5 The anthropologist Leslie Butt (2002) warns us of other dangers that come from a
singular focus on anthropologists of global health as protagonists in the fight for
justice.

6 The anthropologist Tanya Jakimow (2020, 2022) has done an excellent job of
situating affect within the development industry, including an informative focus
on relations to self. Nonetheless, her work demonstrates this subordination of the
intimate to the structural, as her interest in affect is focused on its role as a tool in
larger power relations.

7   Notably, this DIY phenomenon is not restricted to the domain of global health but has been remarked on more widely in connection to development and aid (Develtere & De Bruyn, 2009; Fechter & Schwittay, 2019; McLennan, 2017). I discuss DIY global health more thoroughly in chapter 1.

8   Many of the criteria I discuss are described by the sociologist Judith Lasker (2016) as facets of medical volunteering. The global health scholar Pavinarmatha Ketheeswaran (2015) attempts an empirical account of STMM characteristics and cautions that academic literatures may not accurately capture what is actually going on.

9   This may not be true for all jornadas in Guatemala, and I heard that more specialized surgical jornadas in the cities provided a nominal fee to surgeons for their work, though I was never able to confirm this.

10  Examinations of volunteering around the world demonstrate how religion and culture shape motivations, goals, expectations, and actions (Bornstein, 2012; Mittermaier, 2014, 2019). The volunteers in this research hail from North America. I use the term "Western" to emphasize Eurocentric thinking that translates into volunteers typically finding commonplace what Fassin (2011) refers to as "humanitarian reason."

11  Likewise, the anthropologist Anne-Meike Fechter (2019) argues that these feelings of connection are important for development aid workers.

12  My focus in this introduction is to attend to the "self" in volunteering. However, scholars have productively related volunteering to the state. Muehlebach and Adams view volunteering as the responsibility for caring being transferred from the state onto individual citizens. From this perspective, volunteering is a harbinger of a state being weakened by neoliberal policy. The sociologist Nina Eliasoph (2013) also examines the relationship between volunteering and states but contends that volunteering strengthens the state. She contextualizes volunteering as part of the engagement necessary for democracy.

13  Aristotle lays out nine specific virtues that an individual should cultivate in *Nicomachean Ethics*; however, I use the idea of a virtuous life more generally. Eventually, Aristotle argued, if one practices enough, acting virtuously will become reflexive or second nature.

14  I include myself in this group.

15  The relative privilege of volunteers has produced many silences in these pages— silences regarding colonialism, imperialism, race, etc. My colleagues have demonstrated how historically informed inequities are in fact an incredibly important component of medical volunteering as part of a global health experience (Brada, 2011; Murali, 2022; Sullivan, 2018).

16  While my inspiration for visceral ethics emanates from the ethical turn, other strains of anthropology bear similarities to my project or have developed tools needed for it. Most closely would be João Biehl's (2005) innovative work *Vita*, focusing on his relationship with one woman. I admire and have learned from his treatment of himself as ethnographer in this work; theoretically, my book is

balanced much further on the scale of embracing the internal as explanatory. I also mention reflexive and experimental anthropology that has insisted on the importance of considering the strengths and limits of claims to what we know (Behar, 1993, 1996).

17 In Guatemala, the ministry of health is called the Ministerio de Salud Pública y Asistencia Social, which literally translates to the "Ministry of Public Health and Social Assistance."

18 My use of "protagonist" is not unintentional. Perhaps due to my interest in virtue ethics, upon finishing my first draft, I found a leitmotif marking components of a Greek play running throughout this volume.

19 Ferguson is not alone in insisting that we have much to learn even when we unmoor our scholarship from rigorous conceptions of place. In an interrogation of development, Rottenburg (2009) decided to rid his ethnography of the specificities of place so much so that he set it in a fictional country. Such a move, he argues, shifts the reader's focus away from thinking about the violence wrought as the outcomes of mismanagement of particular people and instead allows the focus to settle on "the significance of general structural principles and the contingencies of the mundane practices of the development world" (Rottenburg, 2009:xvii). In other words, Rottenburg removes place from his writing as it helps him argue that the particularities of action observed are heavily dictated by higher-level structures. While I do not necessarily disagree with his choice, theoretically, his approach is antithetical to mine, as I argue that focusing on higher levels as determinant can obscure how particularities of action contribute to the construction of higher levels.

20 Perhaps the most typical example of this is implementation science, an area of research and practice concerned with "translating" evidence into health services programming. Implicit in this model is the idea that "best practices" can travel across time and space; what works in Nairobi works in Nanjing. Writing from within the field, May, Johnson, and Finch (2016) contend that "context is a problem for implementation science." In other words, the specificities of local settings are seemingly irrelevant for implementation science, except when they obstruct it. Even among this group of authors, who encourage more sophisticated approaches that acknowledge the complexity of real-life settings, context is only interesting insofar as it might affect an intervention.

## CHAPTER 1. TRANSFORMATIONS IN GLOBAL HEALTH

1 There are number of issues with the division of countries into categories like "undeveloped" (which depends on ethnocentric, linear theories that view colonial powers as being the most advanced and judge other countries relative to them) or "low resource" (where countries are actually rich in resources but do not profit from that richness due to issues of local and international governance) or "Global South," "Third World," etc. My own choice is to use "low income and low-middle income," abbreviated LMIC to signal this grouping. Though this categorization,

offered by the World Bank, is also fraught, I choose it because it relies on a basic description of average household income. Of course, this categorization is mute about root causes, such as colonization and imperialism, patterning which countries fall into which categories. I use "high-income country" (HIC) when I mean wealthy countries in general, and "Western countries," when referring to colonial and imperial powers. I acknowledge that these terms are problematic, as is my use of relatively recently coined terms to describe the past. I chose this tactic to help simplify histories of development for those who are unfamiliar, as it enabled me to standardize my terms. However, it is important to acknowledge that I am frequently not using terminology that was used by authors of the works or in the times that I am discussing.

2 When Simon was interning there, the Behrhorst clinic would have been the first of its kind to approach primary health care predicated on grassroots notions of community participation and empowerment. Carroll Behrhorst was a US doctor who founded a clinic in Chimaltenago, a Kaqchikel area of Guatemala, in the 1960s. Behrhorst firmly believed that health must be cultivated by working on root causes, such as malnutrition and poverty. This clinic is famous for propagating one of the first community health worker programs, which was lauded by WHO in the 1970s and has since been a resource for developing similar programs in Africa and Asia (Long, 1985; Maupin, 2015).

3 The relative importance of expertise and the irrelevance of clinical practice to international health is creatively summarized by the anthropologists Erica Bornstein and Peter Redfield (2010). They attempt to provide a heuristic to separate three related fields that engaged in addressing health concerns in LMICs: humanitarianism, development (i.e., international health), and human rights. According to their shorthand, you can tell a humanitarian effort by the involvement of doctors, a development effort by the involvement of economists, and a human rights effort by the involvement of lawyers.

4 The case of Cuba's training and use of physicians to gain influence stands as an exception to this discussion (Blue, 2010; Huish & Kirk, 2007; Pérez & Silva, 2019).

5 The United States, specifically, shifted from funding international health through international organizations (like the WHO) to pursuing policy objectives (including health) through international financial institutions like the World Bank (Foley, 2010) and the International Monetary Fund. The United States' preference for working through international financial institutions (IFIs) is directly related to the difference in governance structures between IFIs and international organizations. The governance structure of international organizations like the UN and its related subsidiary branches, such as the WHO, is dominated by one country, one vote. Because the number of LMICs far outweighs the number of HICs, the United States' influence on global affairs can be tempered. However, unlike the governing structure of the UN, IFIs tie the weight of each country's voting power to its financial contributions. The more funding a country provides, the greater influence the country receives to determine policies and programming. Given the

United States' position as a primary contributor to the World Bank and International Monetary fund, the United States has outsized influence in dictating policy, ensuring that any monies directed there (whether from US or other countries' coffers) are used to pursue its own agendas. Not surprisingly, the United States' shift away from funding international organizations and toward international financial institutions weakened major stakeholders in international health, notably compromising the ability of the WHO to lead and coordinate international health activity, as well as to pursue its particular "health for all" agenda (Gish, 1982).

6 The anthropologists James Pfeiffer and Rachel Chapman, as well as their partners, have made major contributions to our understandings of austerity, particularly through a chronicling of health-sector activities in Mozambique (Pfeiffer & Chapman, 2015; Pfeiffer, Gimbel, et al., 2017; Pfeiffer, Montoya, et al., 2010).

7 The end of the Cold War in 1989 created further challenges that stalled the field of "international health." While post–World War II development agendas had been shaped largely by superpower conflict, the fall of the Soviet Union removed the pressing need for the United States to maintain influence through development assistance. Furthermore, it created space for Western countries to reconsider their priorities. The Institute for Health Metrics and Evaluation, based at the University of Washington, documents an all-time low level of development assistance for health in the beginning of the 1990s, primarily due to decreases in US funding (IHME, 2009).

8 Rohloff et al. (2011) document the explosion of health care NGOs in Guatemala. Mark Schuller's (2012) ethnography explores NGO perceptions of inefficient government and their own sector importance in another Latin American country, Haiti.

9 New modes arose to organize an "unruly mélange" of diverse players (Buse & Walt, 1997, 2000). Garrett's (2007) influential analysis details many of the challenges that arose when multiple players attempted to address enduring issues.

10 While this section traces the rise of global health through the debt crisis in LMICs, Muehlebach (2012) reminds us that austerity has also enfranchised new relations in Europe. She inadvertently provides us with a potential rationale for clinically engaged global health travel when she contends that new ethical imperatives for volunteers to provide care can arise where state services have been withdrawn due to neoliberal austerity. Keshavjee (2014) provides an excellent overview of how this transition to global health was used to spread neoliberal ideology more generally.

11 By "comprehensive primary care," I am referring to a system in which patients have a first point of contact where they can get access to a wide suite of resources needed to maintain their overall health, including health promotion, preventive care, curative care, and rehabilitative care marked by continuity (rather than fragmentation).

12 To be clear, while Koplan et al.'s definition has been influential among "doers" in the global health domain, it has not been taken up among critical global health

scholars. Indeed, what "global health" actually is in the world and its usefulness to scholarship continue to be extraordinarily contentious in critical scholarship (Biehl, 2016; Birn, 2009; Brada, 2023; Fassin, 2012).

13  Notably, my research focuses on licensed clinicians who go abroad, many of whom were surgeons. In many ways, my research reflects some of the best-case scenarios. Many of the people who get involved in global health work or short-term global health placements actually have little to no (medical) skills (Lasker, 2016). Sullivan (2018) documents some of the dangers of unskilled volunteers believing that they have a right to intervene or that their medical interventions are helpful.

14  For more on this claim, see Birn, Pillay, & Holtz, 2009.

15  I use the term "missionaries" to refer to people involved with Christian missions. I use the term "missioner" to refer to people involved with short-term medical missions.

16  In an examination of short-term medical volunteering in Sierra Leone, Srinidhi Murali (2022) contends that contemporary practices continue to mirror colonial practices.

17  Many organizations, such as Faith in Practice, which supply low- to no-cost medicines for medical missions, are openly religious. Notably, Rowthorn et al. (2019) argue that one of the areas where short-term global health experiences are most likely to be legally transgressive is around the import and distribution of medicines.

18  The language of "saving" was prescient, as Philippe came to understand.

19  Many different factors contributed to how each STMM decided what services to offer. The surgical equipment available on-site, past types of demand seen in a patient population, or grants from a sponsoring organization are all examples of factors that could be prioritized to determine what type of professional/specialist was recruited for a particular jornada.

20  Participants' preference for viewing short-term medical missions as professional activities (rather than religious) is not necessarily novel. Indeed, both Malkki (2015) and Halvorson (2018) address how the theme of professionalism was important to people working in the domain of humanitarian medical aid. Furthermore, the idea of professional expertise has been foundational to characterizing the workforce participating in development activities (Escobar, 1988, 1995), including health development (Mosse, 2011; Pfeiffer, 2003). Nevertheless, despite these continuities, "humanitarianism" and "development" were not words that came up; "global health" was.

21  Most of the medical students did not have the necessary language skills to speak to patients, so their prospects for being able to adequately provide many clinical services would have been low.

22  Coordinated public campaigns against infectious diseases have been at the center of health promotion in Latin America for at least a century and are well documented in multiple disciplinary spheres. The theme of infectious disease versus

modernity and progress is so prevalent that beating it back through public works in a central plotline of one of the most famous Latin American novels, *Love in the Time of Cholera* (García Márquez, 1986). Social scientists and historians have illustrated how tropical medicine targeting infectious diseases has been an important intervention supporting colonialism and imperialism in Latin America (Birn & Solórzano, 1999; Cueto, 1992). Infectious diseases, and more particularly helminths, have been a focus of international health cooperation, and indeed the WHO has been producing technical guidelines for reducing infection since at least the 1980s (World Health Organization, 1987, 2002, 2006, 2011). It is noteworthy that like many vaccination programs, the WHO coordinates pharmaceutical companies' donations of helminthic drugs to support the biannual campaign approach taken by Guatemala (World Health Organization, 2017).

23  Though offering education with medication is probably a better intervention than medication alone, necessary changes in sanitation infrastructure that could end parasitic infection are notably not part of either jornada effort.

24  For what it is worth, my husband got a business card from the leader of the jornada, and we used that information to find the dean of the medical school at the Florida university that sponsored this program. Mustering the decades of academic training and disciplinary breadth that we possessed between the two of us, we wrote an email documenting the actions that we had witnessed that day and why they were harmful and providing information on whom to contact in Guatemala to mitigate the likelihood of these sorts of events happening again. We received a "sorry you feel that way" email from the dean extolling the importance of the jornada program as a learning experience for students and informing us that they would continue as delivered.

25  And after the email from the dean, we neither saw nor heard from them again.

26  While I concentrate here on outlining DIY global health, this phenomenon parallels the rise of what has been called "citizen aid" in humanitarian and development sectors (Develtere & De Bruyn, 2009; Fechter & Schwittay, 2019).

27  Notably, the WHO guidelines for the safe use of anthelmintics are public-health guidelines for at-risk populations. A public-health approach to controlling helminths necessarily unfolds over time, and the Florida jornada would have needed to know when the last dose of anthelmintics was distributed to program its own activities. The Florida jornada's methods are closer to guidelines for individual, clinical treatment. The US Centers for Disease Control guidelines for treating newly arrived refugees suggests routine dosing without confirmation of infection for some refugees. Health Canada's guidelines for clinical treatment, however, suggest one dose at confirmation of infection and a second dose three months later.

28  Notable exceptions to this include Herrick and Brooks (2020), Sullivan (2016, 2018), and Prince (2016) and a plethora of student theses (Atterton, 2021; Callanan, 2018; Casler, 2016; Citrin, 2011; Driese, 2022; Gilchrest, 2021; Ketheeswaran, 2015; Murali, 2022; Rieder, 2016; Wilson, 2019). Nevertheless, searching online syl-

labi for general global health courses reveals a continued concentration on formal global health only.

29  My purpose in drawing this distinction is not to endorse formal global health practice as superior practice in the domain. Anthropologists have been prolific in detailing how the design of formal global health can itself contribute to egregiousness (Heckert, 2018; Keshavjee, 2014; Sullivan, 2017) What is important here is that formal and DIY global health operate on different logistics and presumptions.

30  I have previously illustrated this point with reference to NGOs that support STMMs in Guatemala as the main actors (Berry, 2014). Wendland, Erikson, and Sullivan (2016) illustrate this point with reference to medical schools and medical students in the global health domain.

CHAPTER 2. GLOBAL HEALTH AS PROFOUNDLY PERSONAL

1  The message is so ubiquitous that, walking from my university office to the water fountain, I am regaled by posters encouraging students to make a difference, to give back, to go to India or Ecuador, and to work with people who need them.

2  As Keane's main goal in proposing affordances is to provide a synthetic account that can join the "natural" and "social" worlds, he strategically streamlines facets of his argument to center attention on his main goal. Part of this streamlining is evident in the examples of the natural world, which are inevitably inanimate objects (rocks, chairs, etc.). My interpretation is much looser, and I look for instances when volunteers are inspired by things that they perceive as a facet of the external world but not necessarily an object of the natural world.

3  As a translator, I directly interpret the words of each person so that they are understood. I do not give advice or inject myself, my perspectives, or my experiences into the interaction.

4  Given the discrimination and racism against Indigenous people, Carmen might have found it uncomfortable for someone to suggest that she was Indigenous.

5  Obviously race and ethnicity are complex, particularly in Guatemala. Hale (2006) explores a more contemporary understanding of identity allegiance in relation to being Mayan in Guatemala. Paredes (2017) argues that skin color remains important to ethnic hierarchy and identity.

6  My focus in this interaction is on Matthew as what Enfield calls the "perceiving and acting entity." Nevertheless, McDermott and Tylbor (1995:218) remind us that "participation in any social scene requires minimum consensus on what is getting done in the scene." In other words, Carmen's role is just as important to establishing conversational dynamics as Matthew's. While Matthew remains ignorant to who Carmen is, ultimately, Carmen lets Matthew pretend. Finally, I note my own complicity in not correcting Matthew, as well as the importance of my own (potentially flawed) perceptions in recounting these events. Similarly, as this analysis is about how Matthew perceives race, alternate perspectives and critiques of Matthew's perspective are included only insomuch as they help us understand

this interaction. Ironically, how Matthew gets "race" wrong in this interaction provides nice material to demonstrate how race is a social construct that, despite certain similarities, does not travel from context to context.

7 One of the dimensions complicating this section is how volunteers flatten Indigene-ity, poverty, and being Guatemalan. I have pulled one dimension to examine here—that is, Indigeneity—because this is what volunteers talked about most. However, my general impression is consonant with this example: volunteers generally did not have robust knowledge of Guatemala, historically, politically, or socially. I frequently felt slippage, where volunteers assumed that Indigenous, indigent, and Guatema-lan were all interchangeable. This echoes Deomampo (2016), who points out the intertwining of ideologies around "race" and "rescue" that White parents articulate in connection with hiring Indian surrogates—in her case, the parent paying an Indian woman (race) contributes to changing her life (rescue). Deomampo reminds us that, in transnational practice, like STMMs, volunteers' ideologies of race are constructed with already-existing global dynamics that class Guatemalans, and particularly Indigenous Guatemalans, as poor (or poorer).

8 Matthew's response is all the more remarkable when we consider Dana-Ain Davis's (2019) contention that the medical practitioners she writes about in the US viewed racializing their patients as negative (discriminatory) and preferred to view their domain of practice as being "post-racial."

9 Phil was not alone in this sentiment. Another volunteer whom I interviewed had switched jornadas because the patients were not "appropriate." He explained that he was very frustrated during a surgical mission in Antigua when he found out that he had operated on an architect from Guatemala City "who could well afford [private surgery]."

10 It is also worth noting that it is not feasible to screen people for being poor. Just like in North America, it would be difficult to know if someone could afford to pay for care (i.e., was not poor) just by looking at them. Indeed, a foundation-run hospital in Sololá that offered care on a sliding scale employed a phalanx of social workers whose job was to determine how much a family could pay. Visiting a patient at home and interviewing their neighbors was an important component of verifying their financial solubility. Because determining how much a family could pay was so labor-intensive, the hospital only offered sliding fees for patients living in the same town as the hospital.

## CHAPTER 3. TRANSFORMATIVE MOMENTS

1 From a North American medical perspective, this might be a transgression of Antonia's privacy, and I have never seen something like this happen to me nor others in the US or Canada. Nevertheless, notions of privacy, including how they relate to bioethics, are bound to time and place (Goldim & Gibbon, 2015), and I personally did not see this incident creating discomfort for Guatemalans present (or for other jornada volunteers). I previously had a somewhat similar experience accompanying a Kaqchikel woman to a local hospital to have her ovarian cysts

removed. When the surgery was completed and the patient was in post-op waking up from anesthesia, the surgeon came to find us—her family and friends—so that he could show us the cysts, floating in a recycled food jar full of transparent liquid. Another friend shared with me an experience of a surgeon bringing out a parasite in a jar to show that they had successfully removed it from a family member. While neither the ovarian cyst nor parasite were passed around like Antonia's flesh at the jornada, perhaps this practice of showing results of surgery was not so out of place in Guatemala.

2  Notably, Mattingly (2012) provides a complementary argument in her critique of Foucault. Jones (2011, 74), for her part, invents the term "network standard body," derived from the "unaccented 'everyman' network-standard English spoken by news anchors" to highlight this generic actor.

3  "Telephone" is a game of (mis)communication: First, a group of players get in a line. Then, the last person in line whispers a message into the ear of the person directly in front of them, low enough so that none of the other players can hear. That person then whispers what they heard to the person in front of them and so on until the message makes its way up to the player in the front of the line. The last player then says the message aloud for everyone to hear. The game is entertaining because normally the message that the final player recites is only tangentially related to the original message that started the game.

4  The anthropologist Lydia Dixon (2020) writes about the difficulty for patients to trust lab results in the Mexican context.

5  Perhaps because of these mission experiences, for a few years after volunteering, I was drawn to YouTube videos in which people put on EnChroma glasses and see color for the first time in their lives. These videos were typically saturated with just enough emotion to remind me what it felt like to witness someone gaining the raw ability to see.

6  While Bornstein works specifically with volunteers, the anthropologist Betsey Brada (2023) outlines the necessity of transformative encounters in the domain of clinical global health. Through ethnography detailing the experiences of young US clinicians completing placements in Botswana's HIV programs, Brada catalogues the alignment between global health, "heroic medicine," and doctors' transformative experiences. While Brada attends to transformation in relation to subject making, in this chapter, I am concerned with the way transformative experiences primed me to recover different knowledge regarding the moral valence of my own actions.

7  I say "theoretically" because needed diagnostics (e.g., a particular test) or therapies (e.g., a medicine) are frequently not available. Patients, therefore, have to go to a private lab or pharmacy for their treatment to be complete. I describe in-depth costs related to free treatment in the hospital in Sololá in Berry, 2010.

8  Driese (2022) provides a critical account of gratitude at jornadas.

9  Explorations of giving "gifts" have contributed to rich theorizing of social reproduction and the identities, exchanges, and economies on which sociality is

founded (Malinowski, 1922; Mauss, 1990; Rubin, 1975). Anthropological analyses have also prioritized the importance of reciprocity, focusing our attention on what a gift engenders in the world, be it a tie to divinity, bad luck, or even national economic development (Stirrat & Henkel, 1997; cf. Derrida, 1992).

10  Interestingly, Bornstein (2012) points out that some forms of Hindu religious giving focus only on how a gift is important to the giver. Attending only to the effects of the gift on the giver does not undermine the moral integrity of the gift in the case she explores.

11  As noted in the introduction, Lasker (2016) found that using and improving skills was sometimes a motivator for global health volunteering.

12  Notably, there is a huge variety of approaches to charging or not charging among STMMs. Organizations that charged patients (because they believe that patients would value the care more or to facilitate sustainability of their activities) pointed out that potential volunteers often criticized or pushed back against this policy.

13  A speculum is a piece of medical equipment that is typically used for a vaginal exam.

## CHAPTER 4. LACK OF CONTEXT

1  Kidder's book was widely read and was a *New York Times* bestseller. In addition, it was popular as a "common book" for many universities (i.e., a book everyone on campus reads in the same year) and for book clubs. Numerous guides exist on the internet for facilitating academic and lay discussions about the book.

2  Please note that I am concentrating here on Tracy Kidder's narrative, which happens to be about Paul Farmer. I am not suggesting that Farmer believed or propagated this narrative. I note the irony of using Farmer as an example in a chapter about lack of attention to context given that what frequently distinguished Farmer's work is attention to context.

3  I loosely follow Keane's (2016) wrangling with the purported difference between ethics and morality to guide lexical choices in this chapter. Drawing on Bernard Williams, Keane (2016:18) posits that "whereas morality deals with such questions as what one should do next, ethics concerns a manner of life." To illustrate this difference using *Mountains beyond Mountains*, we can see that per Kidder, working in global health is part of Paul Farmer's ethics, as Keane uses the term. Working in global health appears to be a cornerstone of Farmer's life as he prioritizes seeking justice for vulnerable others. Yet we have to drill down to particular actions that Farmer has taken in particular times and particular places to judge his morality. In short, "moral" is used in this chapter to signal a more focused examination of the value of a particular action as "right" or "wrong," while ethics is reserved for "manner of life" in general.

4  We can differentiate between an approach to action on general rules and on situated judgments by examining a hypothetical example of one person killing another person. The Christian commandment that "Thou shalt not kill" is a general rule approach to judging this hypothetical incident. Regardless of

the circumstances, when I determine that one person has killed another, that killer has committed a morally reprehensible action. Situated judgments of one person killing another, on the other hand, would consider context and intent. For example, many people find assisting suicide for terminally ill persons to be morally virtuous despite the fact that in these circumstances one person essentially is ending the life of another. In this case, the context (the fact that the person who is dying may be in pain, will inevitably die, and wants some sense of agency over their life) and intent (the dying person consents to death) leads many to view medically assisted death as humane rather than morally reprehensible.

5  In the introduction, I use the term "ideas of place" to refer to the tendency for global health interventions to treat place as a backdrop that lacks the full depth and complexity of a real place. Please refer to the introduction for further elucidation of ideas of place.

6  I would note that Teresa did not share the comradery that so many other volunteers found in doing things together.

7  Sololá is located in the western highlands and lies over two thousand meters above sea level. Relative to Texas (Teresa's other home), it is definitely "up there."

8  I would be fascinated to find out how this occurred. This collaboration had ended by the time I started my field research at the Sololá hospital in the early 2000s. I interviewed two Guatemalan doctors who worked at the hospital when the mission worked there and a US doctor who headed one of the missions that worked at the hospital, but no one was forthcoming about how and why this deal was made. Teresa did tell me that the first time she met any missioners was when she arrived for work at the hospital one morning, and the whole mission group was outside the gates, being refused entry by the guards. Her recounting of that morning speaks to what we learn from Teresa's own story, that there are factions within the hospital and that it is difficult to get everyone to agree.

9  In recounting this story, my Guatemalan interviewees stressed that the volunteers then went out to enjoy themselves, indirectly casting aspersions on medical missions by tying them more to tourism than to patient care.

10  Again, we return to the contention that what feels right in the moment for volunteers might actually be wrong—that is, might endanger the patient.

11  Perhaps this situation is more familiar to clinicians than it is to me. Stef Shuster (2021:1) chronicles various influences on medical decision-making, particularly use of "spidey senses" to determine treatment in new therapeutic areas, like trans medicine.

## CHAPTER 5. WHERE THERE IS NO DOCTOR

1  A full account of this argument is beyond this chapter; nevertheless, I suggest that most STMMs do not travel to places that do not have access to health care or lack the types of professionals who arrive. Sololá is certainly not such a place. Sololá not only boasts a national hospital but has a private hospital and an NGO hospital. It has health posts and numerous private clinics. As we saw in chapter 4,

it also has a burgeoning diagnostic industry. There are examples of missions organized around surgical specialties absent in a country (including in Guatemala; Davis, Than, & Garton, 2014; Abenavoli, 2005; Magee et al., 2012). These missions require a higher level of coordination with host-country health systems.

2  Barrs et al. (2000), Del Rossi et al. (2003), Homøe, Siim, and Bretlau (2008), and Maine et al. (2012) stand as impressive exceptions to this critique, each attempting to follow up with patients more than one year after surgery. Nevertheless, there are many reasons why surgical STMMs in particular need to be able to follow up with their patients. For example, the living and working conditions of many patients who attend STMMs can hamper surgical outcomes. As Gil et al. (2012:2800) point out, difficult working conditions in Central Africa involving "tough physical tasks" cause high numbers of hernias and "early recurrences with large and invalidating hernias." At the most basic level, Sykes (2014:e46) argues that "simply assuming the care provided is safe and has minimal risks is no longer adequate for [STMMs]." McQueen et al. (2010) point out in their survey of international organizations doing surgical care in LMICs that this assumption is still made: only 78 percent track mortality rates, and only 61 percent track infection rates (and given the self-selected sample, the authors suggest that real numbers are much lower).

3  As mentioned earlier, a *huipil* is the embroidered shirt, and a *corte* is the embroidered skirt that many Mayan women wear.

4  Salmen et al. (2022) use this rationale to suggest that the global health community's firm belief that "rigor" is the best tool to guide our global health interventions may instead be an artifact of the illusion of control.

5  I am not suggesting that Heather should have done something different or that what she did was not right, nor am I asserting that her judgment was wrong. I am merely pointing out her reliance on certain parts of the encounter to form her judgment.

6  It bears reminding that volunteers almost uniformly do not have access to this information, a point to which I return in the conclusion.

CONCLUSION

1  I have provided one example (plans for self-care and monitoring) to illustrate structures inherent to STMMs that may systematically impact the quality of care provided to patients. Atterton (2021), however, cautions us against a transparent focus on quality of care as conceptualized by Western clinicians in humanitarian settings. Using Doctors Without Borders as her case study, she argues that inequalities that characterize humanitarian settings can complicate the provision of care (e.g., create the optic that for these poor people, something is better than nothing). She rightly argues that when we focus on an exported notion of quality of care, our attention to the global dynamics of inequalities that produce the humanitarian setting itself are highjacked.

2  This competes with the priority of making sure that everyone who lined up for care at a medical mission can see a doctor.

3  For example, a couple who sought surgical sterilization told me that the female partner had her uterus removed, instead of her tubes tied. Patients who had hysterectomies typically did not know what had been removed (uterus, fallopian tubes, ovaries?). Most could not answer whether the surgery had been vaginal or abdominal.

4  Driese (2022) methodically catalogues risks created for patients at STMMs in Guatemala.

5  The fourth barrier is liability and perceived threats to programs, meaning that unintentional harm may not be recognized because implementers would have to recognize their own liability and/or because recognizing unintentional harms might lead to a decrease of recipients' trust in programming, ultimately resulting in a failure of programming. This barrier seems arguably less applicable (despite still being relevant) because of the ephemeral nature of STMMs.

6  Notably, many difficulties for patients stem from the fact that jornadas function outside of legal/formal systems, as demonstrated by the example of Cuban medical missions that take place in Guatemala. As an interviewee at the Guatemalan College of Physicians and Surgeons (COLMEDEGUA) explained to me, Cuban doctors are technically also not licensed to practice in Guatemala, as they typically have not completed their necessary internships or service or registered with the college. Nevertheless, because of country-to-country agreements, the Guatemalan Ministry of Health placed Cuban doctors at public health posts, clinics, and hospitals. Because Cuban doctors undertake their missions from within the Guatemalan health system, patients who are unintentionally harmed by foreign Cuban doctors would not experience any more difficulty than if they were unintentionally harmed by a Guatemalan doctor.

7  Nor is competent care enough to make an encounter between a health care provider and patient ethical. Alberto Ferreres (2022) further outlines how encounters between surgical volunteers and patients are contextualized by injustice that stems from the "episodic" nature of short-term medical missions. His concerns echo Atterton's (2021) assertions that certain settings can inspire a sense that any care is better than no care. Rowthorn et al. (2019) outline how much STMM practice falls outside of ethical conduct as defined by the WHO.

8  Zientek and Bonnell (2020) adapt protocols from North America to imagine steps that would have to be taken if treatment at an STMM resulted in an unintended harm. While a useful thought exercise, their model depends on robust monitoring and reporting of harms that certainly does not exist in Guatemala (on this point, see Driese, 2022). Addiss and Amon (2019) describe why redressing harms in the context of global health is difficult.

9  Roche and Hall-Clifford (2015) report the same finding.

10 "The meantime" is used to juxtapose a far more inequitable past and ideally equitable futures, in which LMICs independently deploy resources necessary to support the health of their own populations. Positioning one's intervention "in the

meantime" simultaneously continues equity-demoting practices and allies oneself or one's project with the importance of promoting equity.

11  Driese (2022) and Freedman (2018) both provide empirical examples of ways of thinking translating into inequities. Working in two very different domains (Driese in STMMs in Guatemala and Freedman in Greek refugee camps), they demonstrate how the internal assumptions of volunteers can translate into ideas regarding who is a worthy recipient of care as well as volunteers' disappointment in the behaviors and attitudes of those who receive care.

12  We saw this when Matthew (the clinician in chapter 2) derived satisfaction from delivering health care to a woman whom he erroneously assumed was Mayan.

13  Out of the nineteen volunteers I interviewed, two physicians told me that, after reflecting on their experiences, they would never do another medical mission again because it was not contributing to the type of change that they wanted to make. Many missioners who had years of experience gave astute analyses and typologies of interventions across space and time, providing rich rubrics that made sense of their choices of how to engage. Like Teresa from chapter 4, they calibrated their action amid constantly evolving circumstances.

14  Several of the older volunteers whose careers had preceded computers commented on the fact that they felt that they were finally able to practice medicine again, instead of "practicing paperwork." Redfield (2013) documents a similar sentiment regarding the appeal of Doctors Without Borders as providing opportunities to practice "pure medicine."

15  To reiterate, the ability to practice like this in Sololá is not because rules, safeguards, routines, and accountability measures that typify practice in North America do not exist; rather, it is because STMMs are arranged outside of systems of medical practice. Driese (2022) does an excellent job of outlining the (il)legality of STMMs in Guatemala.

16  Notably, Indigenous, Black, and other people of color have called out and fought racism, discrimination, and land and resource theft for centuries. New modes of communication have perhaps heightened the average person's awareness.

17  The Brocher Declaration outlines six key principles that should inform the organization of short-term experiences in global health: (1) mutual partnership with bidirectional input and learning; (2) empowered host-country and community-defined needs and activities; (3) sustainable programs and capacity building; (4) compliance with applicable laws, ethical standards, and code of conduct; (5) humility, cultural sensitivity, and respect for all involved; and (6) accountability for actions.

18  Nor is this the intention of the declaration.

19  Zarowsky, Haddad, and Nguyen (2013) define vulnerability within the global health domain. Unpacking the use of the term in public health in North American, Katz et al. (2020) remind us that when "vague," labeling a group as "vulnerable" can contribute to pathologizing populations and biologizing health inequities. My use of the term here intentionally captures this more problematic valence as it is endemic to the organization of short-term global health engagements.

20 Again, as Driese (2022) notes, most STMMs in Guatemala occur in places that have good access to public and private care. Reaching places characterized by an absence of health resources is difficult. One interviewee told me that they tried serving a remote area but could not justify taking four days of travel for a two-week jornada, as it significantly reduced the number of patients that could be seen. Moreover, remote areas have much fewer resources in general (markets, buildings, restaurants, etc.), making planning and execution more difficult.

21 Driese (2022) reminds us that even hiring someone to take care of bureaucratic work does not mean that it has been done.

22 The dismal alternative is to sequester ourselves in our own corner of academia and talk merely to each other while lamenting that nothing ever changes.

# REFERENCES

Abenavoli, F. (2005). Operation Smile Humanitarian Missions. *Plastic and Reconstructive Surgery, 115*(1), 356–357. https://doi.org/10.1097/01.PRS.0000146085.51120.97.

Abimbola, S., & Pai, M. (2020). Will global health survive its decolonisation? *Lancet, 396*(10263), 1627–1628. https://doi.org/10.1016/S0140-6736(20)32417-X.

Abramowitz, S., & Panter-Brick, C. (2015). Bringing life into relief: Comparative ethnographies of humanitarian practice. In S. Abramowitz & C. Panter-Brick (Eds.), *Medical humanitarianism: Ethnographies of practice* (Vol. 1, pp. 1–22). Philadelphia: University of Pennsylvania Press.

Adam, T., & de Savigny, D. (2012). Systems thinking for strengthening health systems in LMICs: Need for a paradigm shift. *Health Policy and Planning, 27*(suppl_4), iv1–iv3. https://doi.org/10.1093/heapol/czs084.

Adams, V. (2013a). Evidence-based global public health: Subjects, profits, erasures. In J. Biehl & A. Petryna (Eds.), *When people come first: Critical studies in global health* (pp. 54–90). Princeton, NJ: Princeton University Press.

Adams, V. (2013b). *Markets of sorrow, labors of faith: New Orleans in the wake of Katrina.* Durham, NC: Duke University Press.

Adams, V. (2016). Metrics of the global sovereign: Numbers and stories in global health. In V. Adams (Ed.), *Metrics: What counts in global health* (pp. 21–68). Durham, NC: Duke University Press.

Addiss, D. G., & Amon, J. J. (2019). Apology and Unintended Harm in Global Health. *Health and Human Rights Journal, 21*(1), 19–32.

Allen, T. (2015). Life beyond the bubbles: Cognitive dissonance and humanitarian impunity in Northern Uganda. In S. Abramowitz & C. Panter-Brick (Eds.), *Medical humanitarianism: Ethnographies of practice* (pp. 96–118). Philadelphia: University of Pennsylvania Press.

Amoruso, C., Fuoti, M., Miceli, V., Zito, E., Celano, M. R., De Giorgi, A., & Nebbia, G. (2009). Acute hepatitis as a side effect of albendazole: A pediatric case. *La pediatria medica e chirurgica: Medical and Surgical Pediatrics, 31*(4), 176–178. http://europepmc.org.

Anderson, C. (2016). *White rage: The unspoken truth of our racial divide.* New York: Bloomsbury.

Anderson, T. J., Zizza, C. A., Leche, G. M., Scott, M. E., & Solomons, N. W. (1993). The distribution of intestinal helminth infections in a rural village in Guatemala. *Memorias do Instituto Oswaldo Cruz, 88*, 53–65.

Asgary, R., & Junck, E. (2013). New trends of short-term humanitarian medical volunteerism: Professional and ethical considerations. *Journal of Medical Ethics, 39*(10), 625–631. https://doi.org/10.1136/medethics-2011-100488.

Atterton, C. B. (2021). *Quality care in unequal landscapes: The meanings of quality healthcare in humanitarian settings* [Unpublished doctoral dissertation]. University of Manchester.

Austin, J. L. (1962). *How to do things with words.* Cambridge, MA: Harvard University Press.

Bandyopadhyay, R. (2019). Volunteer tourism and "the white man's burden": Globalization of suffering, white savior complex, religion and modernity. *Journal of Sustainable Tourism, 27*(3), 327–343. https://doi.org/10.1080/09669582.2019.1578361.

Banks, N., & Hulme, D. (2012). *The role of NGOs and civil society in development and poverty reduction.* Brooks World Poverty Institute Working Paper No. 171.

Barnett, R. (2012). *The book of gin: A spirited world history from alchemists' stills and colonial outposts to gin palaces, bathtub gin, and artisanal cocktails.* New York: Grove/Atlantic.

Barrs, D. M., Muller, S. P., Worrndell, D. B., & Weidmann, E. W. (2000). Results of a humanitarian otologic and audiologic project performed outside of the United States: Lessons learned from the "Oye, Amigos!" project. *Otolaryngology—Head and Neck Surgery, 123*(6), 722–727. https://doi.org/10.1067/mhn.2000.110959.

Bauman, Z. (1988). *Freedom.* Milton Keynes, UK: Open University Press.

Beck, E. (2017). *How development projects persist: Everyday negotiations with Guatemalan NGOs.* Durham, NC: Duke University Press.

Behar, R. (1993). *Translated woman: Crossing the border with Esperanza's story.* Boston: Beacon.

Behar, R. (1996). *The vulnerable observer: Anthropology that breaks your heart.* Boston: Beacon.

Belinson, J., Pretorius, R., Zhang, W., Wu, L., Qiao, Y., & Elson, P. (2001). Cervical cancer screening by simple visual inspection after acetic acid. *Obstetrics & Gynecology, 98*(3), 441–444. https://doi.org/10.1016/S0029-7844(01)01454-5.

Ben Fredj, N., Chaabane, A., Chadly, Z., Ben Fadhel, N., Boughattas, N. A., & Aouam, K. (2014). Albendazole-induced associated acute hepatitis and bicytopenia. *Scandinavian Journal of Infectious Diseases, 46*(2), 149–151. https://doi.org/10.3109/003655 48.2013.835068.

Benton, A. (2015). *HIV exceptionalism: Development through disease in Sierra Leone.* Minneapolis: University of Minnesota Press.

Berry, N. S. (2006). Kaqchikel midwives, home births, and emergency obstetric referrals in Guatemala: Contextualizing the choice to stay at home. *Social Science & Medicine, 62*(8), 1958–1969.

Berry, N. S. (2008a). Making pregnancy safer for women around the world: The example of safe motherhood and maternal death in Guatemala. In R. Hahn & M. C. Inhorn (Eds.), *Anthropology and public health: Bridging differences in culture and society* (Vol. 2, pp. 422–446). Oxford: Oxford University Press.

Berry, N. S. (2008b). Who's judging the quality of care? Indigenous Maya and the problem of "not being attended." *Medical Anthropology, 27*(2), 164–189.

Berry, N. S. (2010). *Unsafe motherhood: Mayan maternal mortality and subjectivity in post-war Guatemala* (Vol. 21). New York: Berghahn Books.

Berry, N. S. (2014). Did we do good? NGOs, conflicts of interest and the evaluation of short-term medical missions in Sololá, Guatemala. *Social Science & Medicine, 120,* 344–351.

Biehl, J. (2005). *Vita: Life in a zone of social abandonment.* Berkeley: University of California Press.

Biehl, J. (2016). Theorizing global health. *Medicine Anthropology Theory, 3*(2), 127–142.

Biehl, J., & Petryna, A. (Eds.). (2013). *When people come first: Critical studies in global health.* Princeton, NJ: Princeton University Press.

Birn, A.-E. (2009). The stages of international (global) health: Histories of success or successes of history? *Global Public Health, 4*(1), 50–68.

Birn, A.-E., & Krementsov, N. (2018). "Socialising" primary care? The Soviet Union, WHO and the 1978 Alma-Ata Conference. *BMJ Global Health, 3*(Suppl. 3), e000992. https://doi.org/10.1136/bmjgh-2018-000992.

Birn, A.-E., Pillay, Y., & Holtz, T. H. (2009). *Textbook of international health: Global health in a dynamic world.* Oxford: Oxford University Press.

Birn, A.-E., & Solórzano, A. (1999). Public health policy paradoxes: Science and politics in the Rockefeller Foundation's hookworm campaign in Mexico in the 1920s. *Social Science & Medicine, 49*(9), 1197–1213.

Biruk, C. (2018). *Cooking data: Culture and politics in an African research world.* Durham, NC: Duke University Press.

Blue, S. A. (2010). Cuban medical internationalism: Domestic and international impacts. *Journal of Latin American Geography, 9*(1), 31–49.

Bornstein, E. (2012). *Disquieting gifts: Humanitarianism in New Delhi.* Stanford, CA: Stanford University Press.

Bornstein, E., & Redfield, P. (2010). *Forces of compassion: Humanitarianism between ethics and politics.* Santa Fe, NM: School for Advanced Research Press.

Borovoy, A., & Hine, J. (2008). Managing the unmanageable: Elderly Russian Jewish émigrés and the biomedical culture of diabetes care. *Medical Anthropology Quarterly, 22*(1), 1–26. http://dx.doi.org/10.1111/j.1548-1387.2008.00001.x.

Brada, B. B. (2011). "Not here": Making the spaces and subjects of "global health" in Botswana. *Culture, Medicine, and Psychiatry, 35*(2), 285–312. https://doi.org/10.1007/s11013-011-9209-z.

Brada, B. B. (2016). The contingency of humanitarianism: Moral authority in an African HIV clinic. *American Anthropologist, 118*(4), 755–771. https://doi.org/10.1111/aman.12692.

Brada, B. B. (2023). *Learning to save the world: Global health pedagogies and fantasies of transformation in Botswana.* Ithaca, NY: Cornell University Press.

Brown, H. (2015). Global health partnerships, governance, and sovereign responsibility in western Kenya. *American Ethnologist, 42*(2), 340–355. https://doi.org/10.1111/amet.12134.

Brown, T. M., Cueto, M., & Fee, E. (2006). The World Health Organization and the transition from "international" to "global" public health. *American Journal of Public Health, 96*(1), 62–72. https://doi.org/10.2105/ajph.2004.050831.

Buse, K., & Walt, G. (1997). An unruly mélange? Coordinating external resources to the health sector: A review. *Social Science & Medicine, 45*(3), 449–463.

Buse, K., & Walt, G. (2000). Global public-private partnerships: Part I—a new development in health? *Bulletin of the World Health Organization, 78*, 549–561.

Butt, L. (2002). The suffering stranger: Medical anthropology and international morality. *Medical Anthropology, 21*(1), 1–24. https://doi.org/10.1080/01459740210619.

Callanan, M. I. (2018). *Doctor's orders: A grounded theory of physician power relations in the practice of medicine* [Unpublished doctoral dissertation]. George Washington University.

Casler, J. J. (2016). *Short-term medical missions in urban Nicaraguan healthcare systems: An ethnography of patient use and a social network analysis of integration* [Unpublished doctoral dissertation]. University of Florida. https://search.ebscohost.com.

Chary, A. N., & Flood, D. (2021). Iatrogenic trainwrecks and moral injury. *Anthropology & Medicine, 28*(2), 223–238. https://doi.org/10.1080/13648470.2021.1929831.

Chary, A. N., Messmer, S., Sorenson, E., Henretty, N., Dasgupta, S., & Rohloff, P. (2013). The normalization of childhood disease: An ethnographic study of child malnutrition in rural Guatemala. *Human Organization, 72*(2), 87–97. https://doi.org/10.17730/humo.72.2.f201421074270212.

Chary, A. N., & Rohloff, P. J. (2014). Major challenges to scale up of visual inspection-based cervical cancer prevention programs: The experience of Guatemalan NGOs. *Global Health: Science and Practice, 2*(3), 307–317. https://doi.org/10.9745/ghsp-d-14-00073.

Chi, B. K., Rasch, V., Thị Thúy Hạnh, N., & Gammeltoft, T. (2011). Pregnancy decision-making among HIV positive women in Northern Vietnam: Reconsidering reproductive choice. *Anthropology & Medicine, 18*(3), 315–326. https://doi.org/10.1080/13648470.2011.615909.

Citrin, D. M. (2010). The anatomy of ephemeral care: Health, hunger, and short-term humanitarian intervention in Northwest Nepal. *Studies in Nepali History and Society 15*(1), 27–72.

Citrin, D. M. (2011). *"Paul Farmer made me do it": A qualitative study of short-term medical volunteer work in remote Nepal* [Unpublished doctoral dissertation]. University of Washington.

Closser, S. (2010). *Chasing polio in Pakistan: Why the world's largest public health initiative may fail.* Nashville, TN: Vanderbilt University Press.

Cohen, L. (1998). *No aging in India: Alzheimer's, the bad family, and other modern things.* Berkeley: University of California Press.

Cohen-Fournier, S. M., Brass, G., & Kirmayer, L. J. (2021). Decolonizing health care: Challenges of cultural and epistemic pluralism in medical decision-making with Indigenous communities. *Bioethics, 35*(8), 767–778. https://doi.org/10.1111/bioe.12946.

Cole, T. (2012). The white-savior industrial complex. *The Atlantic, 12*(March).

Cornwall, A., and Brock, K. (2005). "What do buzzwords do for development policy? A critical look at 'participation,' 'empowerment' and 'poverty reduction.'" *Third World Quarterly, 26*(7), 1043–1060.

Crane, J. (2010). Unequal "partners": AIDS, academia, and the rise of global health. *Behemoth—A Journal on Civilisation, 3*(3), 78–97.

Crane, J. (2013). *Scrambling for Africa: AIDS, expertise, and the rise of American global health science.* Ithaca, NY: Cornell University Press.

Cueto, M. (1992). Sanitation from above: Yellow fever and foreign intervention in Peru, 1919–1922. *Hispanic American Historical Review, 72*(1), 1–22. https://doi.org/10.2307/2515945.

Das, V. (2010). Engaging the life of the other: Love and everyday life. In M. Lambek (Ed.), *Ordinary ethics: Anthropology, language, and action* (pp. 376–399). New York: Fordham University Press.

Das, V. (2012). Ordinary ethics. In D. Fassin (Ed.), *A companion to moral anthropology* (pp. 133–149). Chichester, UK: Wiley-Blackwell.

Das, V. (2015). What does ordinary ethics look like? In M. Lambek, V. Das, D. Fassin, & W. Keane, *Four lectures on ethics: Anthropological perspectives*, 53–125. London: Hau Books.

Dave, N. N. (2011). Indian and lesbian and what came next: Affect, commensuration, and queer emergences. *American Ethnologist, 38*(4), 650–665. https://doi.org/10.1111/j.1548–1425.2011.01328.x.

Dave, N. N. (2012). *Queer activism in India: A story in the anthropology of ethics.* Durham, NC: Duke University Press.

Davis, D.-A. (2019). *Reproductive injustice: Racism, pregnancy, and premature birth.* New York: New York University Press.

Davis, M. C., Than, K. D., & Garton, H. J. (2014). Cost effectiveness of a short-term pediatric neurosurgical brigade to Guatemala. *World Neurosurgery, 82*(6), 974–979. https://doi.org/10.1016/j.wneu.2014.08.038.

Del Rossi, C., Attanasio, A., Del Curto, S., D'Agostino, S., & De Castro, R. (2003). Treatment of vaginal atresia at a missionary hospital in Bangladesh: Results and followup of 20 cases. *Journal of Urology, 170*(3), 864–866. http://dx.doi.org/10.1097/01.ju.0000081425.66782.c7.

Deomampo, D. (2016). *Transnational reproduction: Race, kinship, and commercial surrogacy in India.* New York: New York University Press.

Derrida, J. (1992). *Given time: I, Counterfeit money.* Chicago: University of Chicago Press.

Develtere, P., & De Bruyn, T. (2009). The emergence of a fourth pillar in development aid. *Development in Practice, 19*(7), 912–922. https://doi.org/10.1080/09614520903122378.

Dixon, L. Z. (2020). *Delivering health: Midwifery and development in Mexico.* Nashville, TN: Vanderbilt University Press.

Drain, P. K., Primack, A., Hunt, D. D., Fawzi, W. W., Holmes, K. K., & Gardner, P. (2007). Global health in medical education: A call for more training and opportunities. *Academic Medicine, 82*(3), 226–230. https://doi.org/10.1097/ACM.0b013e3180305cf9.

Dressler, W. W., Oths, K. S., & Gravlee, C. C. (2005). Race and ethnicity in public health research: Models to explain health disparities. *Annual Review of Anthropology, 34*, 231–252.

Driese, M. C. (2022). *Short-term medical missions to Guatemala: The preparation, organization and execution of STMMs under the enduring influence of neoliberalism* [Unpublished doctoral dissertation]. Arizona State University.

Eliasoph, N. (2013). *The politics of volunteering.* Cambridge, UK: Polity.

Enfield, N. J. (2011). Sources of asymmetry in human interaction: Enchrony, status, knowledge and agency. In J. Steensing, L. Mondada, & T. Stivers (Eds.), *The morality of knowledge in conversation,* 285–312. Cambridge: Cambridge University Press.

Escobar, A. (1988). Power and visibility: Development and the invention and management of the Third World. *Cultural Anthropology, 3*(4), 428–443. www.jstor.org.

Escobar, A. (1995). *Encountering development: The making and unmaking of the Third World.* Princeton, NJ: Princeton University Press.

Fan, E. (2021). *Commodities of care: The business of HIV testing in China.* Minneapolis: University of Minnesota Press.

Fassin, D. (2011). *Humanitarian reason: A moral history of the present.* Berkeley: University of California Press.

Fassin, D. (2012). That obscure object of global health. In M. C. Inhorn & E. A. Wentzell (Eds.), *Medical anthropology at the intersections histories, activisms, and futures* (pp. 95–115). Durham, NC: Duke University Press.

Fechter, A.-M. (2019). Development and the search for connection. *Third World Quarterly, 40*(10), 1816–1831. https://doi.org/10.1080/01436597.2019.1649089.

Fechter, A.-M., & Schwittay, A. (2019). Citizen aid: Grassroots interventions in development and humanitarianism. *Third World Quarterly, 40*(10), 1769–1780. https://doi.org/10.1080/01436597.2019.1656062.

Ferguson, J. (2006). *Global shadows: Africa in the neoliberal world order.* Durham, NC: Duke University Press.

Ferreres, A. R. (2022). The ethics of medical missions (Con). In V. A. Lonchyna, P. Kelley, & P. Angelos (Eds.), *Difficult decisions in surgical ethics: An evidence-based approach* (pp. 585–598). Cham, Switzerland: Springer.

Ferrinho, P., Van Lerberghe, W., Fronteira, I., Hipólito, F., & Biscaia, A. (2004). Dual practice in the health sector: Review of the evidence. *Human Resources for Health, 2*(1), 14. https://doi.org/10.1186/1478-4491-2-14.

Finkler, K. (1994). *Women in pain: Gender and morbidity in Mexico.* Philadelphia: University of Pennsylvania Press.

Fischer, E. F. (2014). *The good life aspiration, dignity, and the anthropology of wellbeing.* Stanford, CA: Stanford University Press.

Flood, D., Chary, A., Austad, K., Coj, M., Lopez, W., & Rohloff, P. (2018). Patient navigation and access to cancer care in Guatemala. *Journal of Global Oncology, 4*, 1–3. https://doi.org/10.1200/jgo.18.00027.

Foley, E. E. (2008). Neoliberal reform and health dilemmas. *Medical Anthropology Quarterly, 22*(3), 257–273. https://doi.org/10.1111/j.1548-1387.2008.00025.x.

Foley, E. E. (2010). *Your pocket is what cures you: The politics of health in Senegal.* New Brunswick, NJ: Rutgers University Press.

Freedman, J. (2018). Amateur humanitarianism, social solidarity and "volunteer tourism" in the EU refugee "crisis." In A. Ahmad & J. Smith (Eds.), *Humanitarian action and ethics* (pp. 94–111). London: Zed Books.

Gammeltoft, T., & Nguyên, H. T. T. (2007). The commodification of obstetric ultrasound scanning in Hanoi, Viet Nam. *Reproductive Health Matters, 15*(29), 163–171.

García Márquez, G. (1986). *El amor en los tiempos del colera* (6th ed.). Buenos Aires: Editorial Sudamericana.

Garrett, L. (2007). The challenge of global health. *Foreign Affairs*, January–February, pp. 14–38.

Gautier, L., Karambé, Y., Dossou, J.-P., & Samb, O. M. (2022). Rethinking development interventions through the lens of decoloniality in sub-Saharan Africa: The case of global health. *Global Public Health, 17*(2), 180–193. https://doi.org/10.1080/17441692.2020.1858134.

Gil, J., Rodríguez, J. M., Hernández, Q., Gil, E., Balsalobre, M. D., González, M., Torregrosa, N., Verdú, T., Alcaráz, M., & Parrilla, P. (2012). Do hernia operations in African international cooperation programmes provide good quality? *World Journal of Surgery, 36*(12), 2795–2801.

Gilchrest, I. S. (2021). *Contemporary medical missions and iatrogenic violence in Honduras* [Unpublished doctoral dissertation]. American University.

Gish, O. (1982). Selective primary health care: Old wine in new bottles. *Social Science and Medicine, 16*, 1049–1063.

Goldim, J. R., & Gibbon, S. (2015). Between personal and relational privacy: Understanding the work of informed consent in cancer genetics in Brazil. *Journal of Community Genetics, 6*(3), 287–293. https://doi.org/10.1007/s12687-015-0234-4.

Grama, A., Aldea, C. O., Burac, L., Delean, D., Bulata, B., Sirbe, C., Duca, E., Boghitoiu, D., Coroleuca, A., & Pop, T. L. (2020). Etiology and outcome of acute liver failure in children—the experience of a single tertiary care hospital from Romania. *Children, 7*(12), 282. www.mdpi.com.

Gravlee, C. (2009). How race becomes biology: Embodiment of social inequality. *American Journal of Physical Anthropology, 139*(1), 47–57. http://dx.doi.org/10.1002/ajpa.20983.

Gravlee, C., & Sweet, E. (2008). Race, ethnicity, and racism in medical anthropology, 1977–2002. *Medical Anthropology Quarterly, 22*(1), 27–51.

Grech, S. (2015). *Disability and poverty in the global South: Renegotiating development in Guatemala.* Cham, Switzerland: Springer.

Green, T., Green, H., Scandlyn, J., & Kestler, A. (2009). Perceptions of short-term medical volunteer work: A qualitative study in Guatemala. *Globalization and Health, 5*(1), 4. https://doi.org/10.1186/1744-8603-5-4.

Greene, J., Basilico, M. T., Kim, H., & Farmer, P. (2013). Colonial medicine and its legacies. In F. Paul, J. Y. Kim, A. Kleinman, & M. Basilico (Eds.), *Reimagining global health: An introduction* (pp. 33–73). Berkeley: University of California Press.

Guatemala. (1985). Constitution of the Republic of Guatemala. www.oas.org.

Hafner, T., & Shiffman, J. (2012). The emergence of global attention to health systems strengthening. *Health Policy and Planning, 28*(1), 41–50. https://doi.org/10.1093/heapol/czs023.

Hale, C. R. (2006). *Más que un Indio = More than an Indian: Racial ambivalence and neoliberal multiculturalism in Guatemala.* Santa Fe, NM: School of American Research Press.

Hall-Clifford, R., & Cook-Deegan, R. (2019). Ethically managing risks in global health fieldwork: Human rights ideals confront real world challenges. *Health and Human Rights Journal, 21*(1), 7–18.

Halvorson, B. (2018). *Conversionary sites: Transforming medical aid and global Christianity from Madagascar to Minnesota.* Chicago: University of Chicago Press.

Halvorson, B. (2020). Reassessing charitable affect: Volunteerism, affect, and ethical practice in a medical aid agency. *Anthropological Quarterly, 93*(2), 151–175.

Haq, C., Rothenberg, D., Gjerde, C., Bobula, J., Wilson, C., Bickley, L., Cardelle, A., & Joseph, A. (2000). New world views: Preparing physicians in training for global health work. *Family Medicine, 32*(8), 566–572.

Hardiman, D. (2006). Introduction. In D. Hardiman (Ed.), *Healing bodies, saving souls: Medical missions in Asia and Africa* (pp. 5–58). Amsterdam: Brill/Rodopi.

Heckert, C. (2018). *Fault lines of care: Gender, HIV, and global health in Bolivia.* New Brunswick, NJ: Rutgers University Press.

Heron, B. (2007). *Desire for development: Whiteness, gender, and the helping imperative.* Waterloo, ON: Wilfrid Laurier University Press.

Herrick, C., & Brooks, A. (2020). Global health volunteering, the Ebola outbreak, and instrumental humanitarianisms in Sierra Leone. *Transactions of the Institute of British Geographers, 45*(2), 362–376. https://doi.org/10.1111/tran.12356.

Ho, K. (2005). Situating global capitalisms: A view from Wall Street investment banks. *Cultural Anthropology, 20*(1), 68–96.

Høg, E. (2014). HIV scale-up in Mozambique: Exceptionalism, normalisation and global health. *Global Public Health, 9*(1–2), 210–223. https://doi.org/10.1080/17441692.2014.881522.

Homøe, P., Siim, C., & Bretlau, P. (2008). Outcome of mobile ear surgery for chronic otitis media in remote areas. *Otolaryngology—Head and Neck Surgery, 139*(1), 55–61. https://doi.org/10.1016/j.otohns.2008.03.014.

Huish, R., & Kirk, J. M. (2007). Cuban medical internationalism and the development of the Latin American School of Medicine. *Latin American Perspectives, 34*(6), 77–92.

IHME (Institute for Health Metrics and Evaluation). (2009). Financing global health 2009: Tracking development assistance for health. Seattle: University of Washington.

Illich, I. (1975). Clinical damage, medical monopoly, the expropriation of health: Three dimensions of iatrogenic tort. *Journal of medical ethics, 1*(2), 78.

Izadnegahdar, R., Correia, S., Ohata, B., Kittler, A., ter Kuile, S., Vaillancourt, S., Saba, N., & Brewer, T. F. (2008). Global health in Canadian medical education: Current practices and opportunities. *Academic Medicine, 83*(2), 192–198.

Jakimow, T. (2020). *Susceptibility in development: Micropolitics of local development in India and Indonesia.* Oxford: Oxford University Press.

Jakimow, T. (2022). Understanding power in development studies through emotion and affect: Promising lines of enquiry. *Third World Quarterly, 43*(3), 513–524. https://doi.org/10.1080/01436597.2022.2039065.

Janes, C. R., & Corbett, K. K. (2009). Anthropology and global health. *Annual Review of Anthropology, 38*(1), 167–183. https://doi.org/10.1146/annurev-anthro-091908-164314.

Janzen, J. M. (1978). *The quest for therapy in Lower Zaire.* Berkeley: University of California Press.

Jézéquel, J.-H. (2015). Staging a "medical coup"? Médecins Sans Frontières and the 2005 food crisis in Niger. In S. Abramowitz & C. Panter-Brick (Eds.), *Medical humanitarianism: Ethnographies of practice* (pp. 119–135). Philadelphia: University of Pennsylvania Press.

Ji, R., & Cheng, Y. (2021). Thinking global health from the perspective of anthropology. *Global Health Research and Policy, 6*(1), 47. https://doi.org/10.1186/s41256-021-00233-z.

Jobson, R. C. (2018). Road work: Highways and hegemony in Trinidad and Tobago. *Journal of Latin American and Caribbean Anthropology, 23*(3), 457–477. https://doi.org/10.1111/jlca.12345.

Jones, N. L. (2011). Embodied ethics: From the body as specimen and spectacle to the body as patient. In F. E. Mascia-Lees (Ed.), *A companion to the anthropology of the body and embodiment* (pp. 72–85). Oxford, UK: Blackwell.

Jones, R., Crowshoe, L., Reid, P., Calam, B., Curtis, E., Green, M., Huria, T., et al. (2019). Educating for indigenous health equity: An international consensus statement. *Academic Medicine, 94*(4), 512.

Justice, J. (2000). The politics of child survival. In I. M. Whiteford & L. Manderson (Eds.), *Global health policy, local realities: The fallacy of the level playing field* (pp. 23–38). Boulder, CO: Lynne Rienner.

Kalofonos, I. (2021). *All I eat is medicine: Going hungry in Mozambique's AIDS economy.* Berkeley: University of California Press.

Kamat, V. R. (2013). *Silent violence: Global health, malaria, and child survival in Tanzania.* Tucson: University of Arizona Press.

Katz, A. S., Hardy, B.-J., Firestone, M., Lofters, A., & Morton-Ninomiya, M. E. (2020). Vagueness, power and public health: Use of "vulnerable" in public health literature. *Critical Public Health, 30*(5), 601–611. https://doi.org/10.1080/09581596.2019.1656800.

Keane, W. (2014a). Affordances and reflexivity in ethical life: An ethnographic stance. *Anthropological Theory, 14*(1), 3–26. https://doi.org/10.1177/1463499614521721.

Keane, W. (2014b). Freedom, reflexivity, and the sheer everydayness of ethics. *HAU: Journal of Ethnographic Theory, 4*(1), 443–457. https://doi.org/10.14318/hau4.1.027.

Keane, W. (2016). *Ethical life: Its natural and social histories.* Princeton, NJ: Princeton University Press.

Kendi, I. X. (2019). *How to be an antiracist.* New York: Random House.

Kenworthy, N. J., & Parker, R. (2014). HIV scale-up and the politics of global health. *Global Public Health, 9*(1–2), 1–6.

Keshavjee, S. (2014). *Blind spot: How neoliberalism infiltrated global health.* Berkeley: University of California Press.

Ketheeswaran, P. (2015). *Good intentions with unknown consequences: Understanding short term medical missions* [Unpublished master's thesis]. Boston University.

Khalid, H., & Martin, E. G. (2019). Relationship between network operators and risky sex behaviors among female versus transgender commercial sex workers in Pakistan. *AIDS Care, 31*(6), 767–776. https://doi.org/10.1080/09540121.2018.1557317.

Khan, M., Abimbola, S., Aloudat, T., Capobianco, E., Hawkes, S., & Rahman-Shepherd, A. (2021). Decolonising global health in 2021: A roadmap to move from rhetoric to reform. *BMJ Global Health, 6*(3), e005604. https://doi.org/10.1136/bmjgh-2021-005604.

Kidder, T. (2003). *Mountains beyond mountains.* New York: Random House.

King, M., Smith, A., & Gracey, M. (2009). Indigenous health part 2: The underlying causes of the health gap. *The Lancet, 374*(9683), 76–85.

King, T. (2017). *The inconvenient Indian illustrated: A curious account of native people in North America.* Toronto: Doubleday Canada.

Kinsbergen, S. (2019). The legitimacy of Dutch do-it-yourself initiatives in Kwale County, Kenya. *Third World Quarterly, 40*(10), 1850–1868. https://doi.org/10.1080/01436597.2019.1644497.

Koplan, J. P., Bond, T. C., Merson, M. H., Reddy, K. S., Rodriguez, M. H., Sewankambo, N. K., & Wasserheit, J. N. (2009). Towards a common definition of global health. *The Lancet, 373*(9679), 1993–1995.

Kwete, X., Tang, K., Chen, L., Ren, R., Chen, Q., Wu, Z., Cai, Y., & Li, H. (2022). Decolonizing global health: What should be the target of this movement and where does it lead us? *Global Health Research and Policy, 7*(1), 3. https://doi.org/10.1186/s41256-022-00237-3.

Laidlaw, J. (2013). *The subject of virtue: An anthropology of ethics and freedom.* Cambridge: Cambridge University Press.

Lambek, M. (2010). *Ordinary ethics: Anthropology, language, and action.* New York: Fordham University Press.

Lasker, J. (2016). *Hoping to help: The promises and pitfalls of global health volunteering.* Ithaca, NY: Cornell University Press.

Lauritz, A. J., Jerry, W. M., David, D. D., & Harold, E. L. (2009). Prevalence of multigastrointestinal infections with helminth, protozoan and Campylobacter spp. in Guatemalan children. *Journal of Infection in Developing Countries, 3*(3). https://doi.org/10.3855/jidc.41.

Leinaweaver, J. B. (2013). Toward an anthropology of ingratitude: Notes from Andean kinship. *Comparative Studies in Society and History, 55*(3), 554–578. https://doi.org/10.1017/S0010417513000248.

Long, W. R. (1985, August 25). A rebirth in Guatemala: As war subsides, U.S. doctor's unique rural health program finds new life. *LA Times.* www.latimes.com.

Lorway, R. (2017). Making global health knowledge: Documents, standards, and evidentiary sovereignty in HIV interventions in South India. *Critical Public Health, 27*(2), 177–192. https://doi.org/10.1080/09581596.2016.1262941.

Lugalla, J. L. P. (1995). The impact of structural adjustment policies on women's and children's health in Tanzania. *Review of African Political Economy, 22*(63), 43–53. https://doi.org/10.1080/03056249508704099.

MacDonald, M. (2017). Why ethnography matters in global health: The case of the traditional birth attendant. *Journal of Global Health, 7*(2), 020302. https://doi.org/10.7189/jogh.07.020302.

Magee, W. P., Raimondi, H. M., Beers, M., & Koech, M. C. (2012). Effectiveness of international surgical program model to build local sustainability. *Plastic Surgery International, 2012,* 185785.

Mahat, A., Citrin, D., & Bista, H. (2018). NGOs, partnerships, and public-private discontent in Nepal's health care sector. *Medicine Anthropology Theory, 5*(2), 100–126.

Mahmood, S. (2005). *Politics of piety: The Islamic revival and the feminist subject.* Princeton, NJ: Princeton University Press.

Maine, R. G., Hoffman, W. Y., Palacios-Martinez, J. H., Corlew, D. S., & Gregory, G. A. (2012). Comparison of fistula rates after palatoplasty for international and local surgeons on surgical missions in Ecuador with Rates at a craniofacial center in the United States. *Plastic and Reconstructive Surgery, 129*(2), 319e–326e 310.1097/PRS.1090b1013e31823aea31827e. http://journals.lww.com.

Malinowski, B. (1922). *Argonauts of the Western Pacific: An account of native enterprise and adventure in the archipelagoes of Melanesian New Guinea.* London: Routledge.

Malkki, L. H. (2015). *The need to help: The domestic arts of international humanitarianism.* Durham, NC: Duke University Press.

Mantey, E. E., Doh, D., Lasker, J. N., Alang, S., Donkor, P., & Aldrink, M. (2021). Ghanaian views of short-term medical missions. The pros, the cons, and the possibilities for improvement. *Globalization and Health, 17*(1), 115. https://doi.org/10.1186/s12992-021-00741-0.

Maractho, E. C., Lasker, J., Alang, S., & Austin, K. (2022). *Enhancing the value of short term volunteer missions in health from host country perspectives: The case of Uganda.* Africa Policy Centre, Uganda Christian University.

Marin Zuluaga, J. I., Marin Castro, A. E., Perez Cadavid, J. C., & Restrepo Gutierrez, J. C. (2013). Albendazole-induced granulomatous hepatitis: A case report. *Journal of Medical Case Reports, 7*(1), 201. https://doi.org/10.1186/1752-1947-7-201.

Marten, M. G., & Sullivan, N. (2020). Hospital side hustles: Funding conundrums and perverse incentives in Tanzania's publicly-funded health sector. *Social Science & Medicine, 244,* 112662. https://doi.org/10.1016/j.socscimed.2019.112662.

Mattingly, C. (2012). Two virtue ethics and the anthropology of morality. *Anthropological Theory, 12*(2), 161–184. https://doi.org/10.1177/1463499612455284.

Mattingly, C. (2014). The moral perils of a superstrong Black mother. *Ethos, 42*(1), 119–138. https://doi.org/10.1111/etho.12042.

Maupin, J. (2009). "Fruit of the accords": Healthcare reform and civil participation in Highland Guatemala. *Social Science & Medicine, 68*(8), 1456–1463. https://doi.org/10.1016/j.socscimed.2009.01.045.

Maupin, J. (2015). Shifting identities. *Annals of Anthropological Practice, 39*(1), 73–88. https://doi.org/10.1111/napa.12065.

Mauss, M. (1990). *The gift: The form and reason for exchange in archaic societies.* New York: Routledge.

May, C. R., Johnson, M., & Finch, T. (2016). Implementation, context and complexity. *Implementation Science, 11*(1), 141. https://doi.org/10.1186/s13012-016-0506-3.

McDermott, R. P., & Tylbor, H. (1995). On the necessity of collusion. In D. Tedlock & B. Mannheim (Eds.), *The dialogic emergence of culture* (pp. 218–236). Urbana: University of Illinois Press.

McKay, R. (2017). *Medicine in the meantime: The work of care in Mozambique.* Durham, NC: Duke University Press.

McLennan, S. J. (2017). Passion, paternalism, and politics: DIY development and independent volunteers in Honduras. *Development in Practice, 27*(6), 880–891.

McQueen, K. K., Hyder, J. A., Taira, B. R., Semer, N., Burkle, F. M., & Casey, K. M. (2010). The provision of surgical care by international organizations in developing countries: A preliminary report. *World Journal of Surgery, 34*(3), 397–402.

Mendez-Dominguez, A., Jose Antonio Aparicio, Q., Arvelo-Jimenez, N., Nelly, A.-J., Batt, C., Bozzoli de Wille, M. E., Dessaint, A. Y., et al. (1975). Big and little traditions in Guatemalan anthropology [and comments and replies]. *Current Anthropology, 16*(4), 541–552. http://www.jstor.org/stable/2741629.

Mishra, A. (2014). "Trust and teamwork matter": Community health workers' experiences in integrated service delivery in India. *Global Public Health, 9*(8), 960–974. https://doi.org/10.1080/17441692.2014.934877.

Mittermaier, A. (2014). Beyond compassion: Islamic voluntarism in Egypt. *American Ethnologist, 41*(3), 518–531. https://doi.org/10.1111/amet.12092.

Mittermaier, A. (2019). *Giving to God: Islamic charity in revolutionary times.* Berkeley: University of California Press.

Mogaka, O. e. F., Stewart, J., & Bukusi, E. (2021). Why and for whom are we decolonising global health? *Lancet Global Health, 9*(10), e1359–e1360. https://doi.org/10.1016/S2214-109X(21)00317-X.

Morrison, T. (2017). *The origin of others.* Cambridge, MA: Harvard University Press.

Mosse, D. (2011). *Adventures in Aidland: The anthropology of professionals in international development.* New York: Berghahn Books.

MSPAS. (2022). MSPAS avanza en la primera jornada de desparasitación 2022. https://prensa.gob.gt.

Muehlebach, A. (2012). *The moral neoliberal: Welfare and citizenship in Italy*. Chicago: University of Chicago Press.

Mumtaz, Z., & Salway, S. (2009). Understanding gendered influences on women's reproductive health in Pakistan: Moving beyond the autonomy paradigm. *Social Science & Medicine, 68*(7), 1349–1356. www.sciencedirect.com.

Murali, S. (2022). *Coloniality in global health: Dependency, medical volunteerism, and maternal mortality* [Special honors thesis]. University of Texas at Austin.

Mussa, A. H., Pfeiffer, J., Gloyd, S. S., & Sherr, K. (2013). Vertical funding, non-governmental organizations, and health system strengthening: perspectives of public sector health workers in Mozambique. *Human Resources for Health, 11*(1), 26. https://doi.org/10.1186/1478-4491-11-26.

Navaro-Yashin, Y. (2009). Affective spaces, melancholic objects: ruination and the production of anthropological knowledge. *Journal of the Royal Anthropological Institute, 15*(1), 1–18. https://doi.org/10.1111/j.1467-9655.2008.01527.x.

Nelson, B. D., Lee, A. C., Newby, P., Chamberlin, M. R., & Huang, C.-C. (2008). Global health training in pediatric residency programs. *Pediatrics, 122*(1), 28–33.

Nelson, D. M. (1999). *A finger in the wound: Body politics in quincentennial Guatemala*. Berkeley: University of California Press.

Newell, S. (2018). The affectiveness of symbols: Materiality, magicality, and the limits of the antisemiotic turn. *Current Anthropology, 59*(1), 1–22. https://doi.org/10.1086/696071.

Ngalamulume, K. (2004). Keeping the city totally clean: Yellow fever and the politics of prevention in colonial Saint-Louis-du-Sènègal, 1850–1914. *Journal of African History, 45*(2), 183–202.

Nguyen, V.-K. (2010). *The republic of therapy: Triage and sovereignty in West Africa's time of AIDS*. Durham, NC: Duke University Press.

Non, A. L., & Gravlee, C. C. (2015). Biology and culture beyond the genome: Race, racism, and health. *American Anthropologist, 117*(4), 737–738.

Nouvet, E. (2016). Extra-ordinary aid and its shadows: The work of gratitude in Nicaraguan humanitarian healthcare. *Critique of Anthropology, 36*(3), 244–263. https://doi.org/10.1177/0308275x16646835.

Nouvet, E., Chan, E., & Schwartz, L. J. (2018). Looking good but doing harm? Perceptions of short-term medical missions in Nicaragua. *Global Public Health, 13*(4), 456–472. https://doi.org/10.1080/17441692.2016.1220610.

Oluo, I. (2019). *So you want to talk about race*. New York: Seal.

Ossome, L. (2015). In search of the state? Neoliberalism and the labour question for pan-African feminism. *Feminist Africa, 20*, 6–25.

Pandian, A. (2009). *Crooked stalks: Cultivating virtue in South India*. Durham, NC: Duke University Press.

Pandian, A., & Ali, D. (2010). *Ethical life in South Asia*. Bloomington: Indiana University Press.

Paredes, C. L. (2017). Mestizaje and the significance of phenotype in Guatemala. *Sociology of Race and Ethnicity, 3*(3), 319–337.

Pérez, J. O., & Silva, A. L. (2019). Cuban medical internationalism through a feminist perspective. *Contexto Internacional, 41*, 65–88.

Pfeiffer, J. (2003). International NGOs and primary health care in Mozambique: The need for a new model of collaboration. *Social Science & Medicine, 56*(4), 725–738.

Pfeiffer, J., & Chapman, R. (2015). An anthropology of aid in Africa. *The Lancet, 385*(9983), 2144–2145. https://doi.org/10.1016/S0140-6736(15)61013-3.

Pfeiffer, J., Gimbel, S., Chilundo, B., Gloyd, S., Chapman, R., & Sherr, K. (2017). Austerity and the "sector-wide approach" to health: The Mozambique experience. *Social Science & Medicine, 187*, 208–216. https://doi.org/10.1016/j.socscimed.2017.05.008.

Pfeiffer, J., Montoya, P., Baptista, A. J., Karagianis, M., Pugas, M. de Morais, Micek, M., Johnson, W., Sherr, K., Gimbel, S., Baird, S., Lambdin, B., & Gloyd, S. (2010). Integration of HIV/AIDS services into African primary health care: lessons learned for health system strengthening in Mozambique—a case study. *Journal of the International AIDS Society, 13*(1), 3–3.

Pfeiffer, J., & Nichter, M. (2008). What can critical medical anthropology contribute to global health? A health systems perspective. *Medical Anthropology Quarterly, 22*(4), 410–415. www.jstor.org.

Pigg, S. L. (2013). On sitting and doing: Ethnography as action in global health. *Social Science & Medicine, 99*, 127–134. https://doi.org/10.1016/j.socscimed.2013.07.018.

Poleykett, B. (2016). Data, desire and recognition: Learning to identify a "prostitute" in Dakar. *Ethnography, 17*(4), 480–496. https://doi.org/10.1177/1466138116641439.

Powis, R. (2022). (Mis)measuring men's involvement in global health: the case of expectant fathers in Dakar, Senegal. *BMC Pregnancy and Childbirth, 22*(1), 754. https://doi.org/10.1186/s12884-022-05093-0.

Prasad, S., Aldrink, M., Compton, B., Lasker, J., Donkor, P., Weakliam, D., Rowthorn, V., et al. (2022). Global health partnerships and the Brocher Declaration: Principles for ethical short-term engagements in global health. *Annals of Global Health, 88*(1).

Prince, R. J. (2016). *Volunteer economies: The politics & ethics of voluntary labour in Africa*. Woodbridge, UK: James Currey.

Prince, R. J., & Otieno, P. (2014). In the shadowlands of global health: Observations from health workers in Kenya. *Global Public Health, 9*(8), 927–945. https://doi.org/10.1080/17441692.2014.941897.

Qureshi, A. (2014). Up-scaling expectations among Pakistan's HIV bureaucrats: Entrepreneurs of the self and job precariousness post-scale-up. *Global Public Health, 9*(1–2), 73–84. https://doi.org/10.1080/17441692.2013.870590.

Rasch, E. D. (2012). Transformations in citizenship: Local resistance against mining projects in Huehuetenango (Guatemala). *Journal of Developing Societies, 28*(2), 159–184. https://doi.org/10.1177/0169796x12448756.

Ravishankar, N., Gubbins, P., Cooley, R. J., Leach-Kemon, K., Michaud, C. M., Jamison, D. T., & Murray, C. J. (2009). Financing of global health: Tracking development assistance for health from 1990 to 2007. *The Lancet, 373*(9681), 2113–2124.

Redfield, P. (2013). *Life in crisis: The ethical journey of doctors without borders*. Berkeley: University of California Press.

Rieder, S. (2016). *Biomedical disenchantments: Practices, discourses, and imaginaries of transnational biomedicalization in rural Ethiopia* [Unpublished doctoral dissertation]. University of Illinois at Urbana-Champaign.

Roche, S., Brockington, M., Fathima, S., Nandi, M., Silverberg, B., Rice, H., & Hall-Clifford, R. (2018). Freedom of choice, expressions of gratitude: Patient experiences of short-term surgical missions in Guatemala. *Social Science & Medicine, 208*, 117–125. https://doi.org/10.1016/j.socscimed.2018.05.021.

Roche, S., & Hall-Clifford, R. (2015). Making surgical missions a joint operation: NGO experiences of visiting surgical teams and the formal health care system in Guatemala. *Global Public Health, 10*(10), 1201–1214. https://doi.org/10.1080/17441692.2015.1011189.

Rohloff, P., Díaz, A. K., & Dasgupta, S. (2011). "Beyond development": A critical appraisal of the emergence of small health care non-governmental organizations in rural Guatemala. *Human Organization, 70*(4), 427–437. www.jstor.org.

Rottenburg, R. (2009). *Far-fetched facts: A parable of development aid.* Cambridge, MA: MIT Press.

Rowthorn, V., Loh, L., Evert, J., Chung, E., & Lasker, J. (2019). Not above the law: A legal and ethical analysis of short-term experiences in global health. *Annals of Global Health, 85*(1).

Rubin, G. (1975). The traffic in women: Notes on the "political economy" of sex. In R. R. Reiter (Ed.), *Toward an Anthropology of Women* (pp. 157–210). New York: Monthly Review Press.

Salmen, C. R., Magerenge, R., Ndunyu, L., & Prasad, S. (2022). Rethinking our rigor mortis: Creating space for more adaptive and inclusive truth-seeking in community-based global health research in Kenya. *Global Public Health, 17*(12), 4002–4013. https://doi.org/10.1080/17441692.2019.1629609.

Samsky, A. (2012). Scientific sovereignty: How international drug donation programs reshape health, disease, and the state. *Cultural Anthropology, 27*(2), 310–332. https://doi.org/10.1111/j.1548-1360.2012.01145.x.

Scheper-Hughes, N., & Lock, M. M. (1987). The mindful body: A prolegomenon to future work in medical anthropology. *Medical Anthropology Quarterly, 1*(1), 6–41. https://doi.org/10.1525/maq.1987.1.1.02a00020.

Schnable, A. (2021). *Amateurs without borders: The aspirations and limits of global compassion.* Berkeley: University of California Press.

Schuller, M. (2012). *Killing with kindness: Haiti, international aid, and NGOs.* New Brunswick, NJ: Rutgers University Press.

Shuster, S. M. (2021). *Trans medicine: The emergence and practice of treating gender.* New York: New York University Press.

Simpson, L. B. (2020). *Noopiming: The cure for white ladies.* Toronto: House of Anansi.

Skoggard, I., & Waterston, A. (2015). Introduction: Toward an anthropology of affect and evocative ethnography. *Anthropology of Consciousness, 26*(2), 109–120. https://doi.org/10.1111/anoc.12041.

Smith-Morris, C., Rodriguez, S., Soto, R., Spencer, M., & Meneghini, L. (2021). De-colonizing care at diagnosis: Culture, history, and family at an urban inter-tribal clinic. *Medical Anthropology Quarterly, 35*(3), 364–385. https://doi.org/10.1111/maq.12645

Sorensen, W., Cappello, M., Bell, D., DiFedele, L., & Brown, M. (2011). Poly-helminth infection in east Guatemalan school children. *Journal of Global Infectious Diseases, 3*(1), 25–31. https://doi.org/10.4103/0974-777x.77292.

Stewart, K. (2007). *Ordinary affects.* Durham, NC: Duke University Press.

Stirrat, R. L., & Henkel, H. (1997). The development gift: The problem of reciprocity in the NGO world. *Annals of the American Academy of Political and Social Science, 554*(1), 66–80. https://doi.org/10.1177/0002716297554001005.

Stodulka, T., Selim, N., & Mattes, D. (2018). Affective scholarship: Doing anthropology with epistemic affects. *Ethos, 46*(4), 519–536. https://doi.org/10.1111/etho.12219.

Storeng, K. T. (2014). The GAVI alliance and the "Gates approach" to health system strengthening. *Global Public Health, 9*(8), 865–879. https://doi.org/10.1080/17441692.2014.940362.

Storeng, K. T., & Béhague, D. P. (2016). "Lives in the balance": The politics of integration in the Partnership for Maternal, Newborn and Child Health. *Health Policy and Planning, 31*(8), 992–1000. https://doi.org/10.1093/heapol/czw023.

Storeng, K. T., Prince, R. J., & Mishra, A. (2018). The politics of health systems strengthening. In R. Parker & J. García (Eds.), *Routledge handbook on the politics of global health* (pp. 114–121). London: Routledge.

Street, A. (2014). *Biomedicine in an unstable place: Infrastructure and personhood in a Papua New Guinean hospital.* Durham, NC: Duke University Press.

Strunz, E. C., Addiss, D. G., Stocks, M. E., Ogden, S., Utzinger, J., & Freeman, M. C. (2014). Water, sanitation, hygiene, and soil-transmitted helminth infection: A systematic review and meta-analysis. *PLOS Medicine, 11*(3), e1001620. https://doi.org/10.1371/journal.pmed.1001620.

Suh, S. (2021). *Dying to count: Post-abortion care and global reproductive health politics in Senegal.* New Brunswick, NJ: Rutgers University Press.

Sullivan, N. (2011). Mediating abundance and scarcity: Implementing an HIV/AIDS-targeted project within a government hospital in Tanzania. *Medical Anthropology, 30*(2), 202–221. https://doi.org/10.1080/01459740.2011.552453.

Sullivan, N. (2016). Hosting gazes: Clinical volunteer tourism & hospital hospitality in Tanzania. In R. P. H. Brown (Ed.), *Volunteer economies: The politics and ethics of voluntary labour in Africa* (pp. 140–163). Rochester, NY: James Currey.

Sullivan, N. (2017). Multiple accountabilities: Development cooperation, transparency, and the politics of unknowing in Tanzania's health sector. *Critical Public Health, 27*(2), 193–204. https://doi.org/10.1080/09581596.2016.1264572.

Sullivan, N. (2018). International clinical volunteering in Tanzania: A postcolonial analysis of a global health business. *Global Public Health, 13*(3), 310–324. https://doi.org/10.1080/17441692.2017.1346695.

Sykes, K. J. (2014). Short-term medical service trips: A systematic review of the evidence. *American Journal of Public Health, 104*(7), e38–e48. https://doi.org/10.2105/AJPH.2014.301983.

Szlezák, N. A., Bloom, B. R., Jamison, D. T., Keusch, G. T., Michaud, C. M., Moon, S., & Clark, W. C. (2010). The global health system: Actors, norms, and expectations in transition. *PLOS Medicine, 7*(1), e1000183. https://doi.org/10.1371/journal.pmed.1000183.

Taylor-Robinson, D. C., Maayan, N., Soares-Weiser, K., Donegan, S., & Garner, P. (2012). Deworming drugs for soil-transmitted intestinal worms in children: Effects on nutritional indicators, haemoglobin and school performance. *Cochrane Database of Systematic Reviews, 11*. https://doi.org/10.1002/14651858.CD000371.pub5.

Tsai, J., Cerdena, J., Khazanchi, R., Lindo, E., Marcelin, J., Rajagopalan, A., Sandoval, R. S., Westby, A., & Gravlee, C. C. (2020). There is no "African American physiology": The fallacy of racial essentialism. *Journal of Internal Medicine, 288*(3), 368–370.

Tsing, A. L. (2005). *Friction: An ethnography of global connection.* Princeton, NJ: Princeton University Press.

Turner, V. (1986). Dewey, Dilthey, and drama: An essay in the anthropology of experience. In V. Turner & E. M. Bruner (Eds.), *The anthropology of experience* (pp. 33–44). Urbana: University of Illinois Press.

Turpel-Lafond, M. E., & Johnson, H. (2021). In plain sight: Addressing Indigenous-specific racism and discrimination in BC health care. *BC Studies: The British Columbian Quarterly, 209*, 7–17.

Turshen, M. (1999). *Privatizing health services in Africa.* New Brunswick, NJ: Rutgers University Press.

Ulysse, G. (2002). Conquering duppies in Kingston: Miss Tiny and me, fieldwork conflicts, and being loved and rescued. *Anthropology and Humanism, 27*(1), 10–26.

Unnithan, M., & Kasstan, B. (2021). "But it's not that they don't love their girls": Gender equality, reproductive rights and sex-selective abortion in Britain. *Medical Anthropology, 41*(6–7), 645–658. https://doi.org/10.1080/01459740.2021.2002857.

Vaughan, M. (1991). *Curing their ills: Colonial power and African illness.* Stanford, CA: Stanford University Press.

Vongsathorn, K. (2012). "First and foremost the evangelist"? Mission and government priorities for the treatment of leprosy in Uganda, 1927–48. *Journal of Eastern African Studies, 6*(3), 544–560. https://doi.org/10.1080/17531055.2012.696906.

Wagner, L. (2015). Compassion and care at the limits of privilege: Haitian doctors amid the influx of foreign humanitarian volunteers. In S. Abramowitz & C. Panter-Brick (Eds.), *Medical humanitarianism: Ethnographies of practice* (pp. 41–57). Philadelphia: University of Pennsylvania Press.

Wendland, C. L. (2012). Moral maps and medical imaginaries: Clinical tourism at Malawi's College of Medicine. *American Anthropologist, 114*(1), 108–122. https://doi.org/10.1111/j.1548-1433.2011.01400.x.

Wendland, C. L., Erikson, S. L., & Sullivan, N. (2016). Moral complexity and rhetorical simplicity in "global health" volunteering. In R. J. Prince & H. Brown (Eds.), *Volunteer economies: The politics and ethics of voluntary labour in Africa* (pp. 164–182). Woodbridge, UK: James Currey.

Werner, D., Thuman, C., & Maxwell, J. (2017). *Where there is no doctor: A village health care handbook* (Rev. ed.). Palo Alto, CA: Hesperian Foundation.

Whyte, S. R. (2002). Subjectivity and subjunctivity: Hoping for health in eastern Uganda. In R. P. Werbner (Ed.), *Postcolonial subjectivities in Africa* (pp. 171–190). London: Zed Books.

Wilson, B. (2019). *An unruly mélange in a postcolonial state: The cultural politics of short-term global health engagements in Dominican Republic bateyes* [Unpublished doctoral dissertation]. University of Texas Medical Branch.

Wilson, B. (2021). When numbers eclipse narratives: A cultural-political critique of the "ethical" impacts of short-term experiences in global health in Dominican Republic bateyes. *Medical Humanities, 48*(2). https://doi.org/10.1136/medhum-2021-012252.

Wojcicki, J. M., & Malala, J. (2001). Condom use, power and HIV/AIDS risk: Sex-workers bargain for survival in Hillbrow/Joubert Park/Berea, Johannesburg. *Social Science & Medicine, 53*(1), 99–121. https://doi.org/10.1016/S0277-9536(00)00315-4.

World Health Organization. (1987). *Prevention and control of intestinal parasitic infections*. Geneva: World Health Organization.

World Health Organization. (2002). *Helminth control in school age children: A guide for managers of control programmes*. Geneva: World Health Organization.

World Health Organization. (2006). *Preventive chemotherapy in human helminthiasis: Coordinated use of anthelminthic drugs in control interventions: A manual for health professionals and programme managers*. Geneva: World Health Organization.

World Health Organization. (2007). *Everybody's business—strengthening health systems to improve health outcomes: WHO's framework for action* (9241596074). Geneva: World Health Organization.

World Health Organization. (2011). *Helminth control in school age children: A guide for managers of control programmes* (2nd ed.) Geneva: World Health Organization.

World Health Organization. (2017). *Guideline: Preventive chemotherapy to control soil-transmitted helminth infections in at-risk population groups*. Geneva: World Health Organization.

Yates-Doerr, E. (2015). *The weight of obesity: Hunger and global health in postwar Guatemala*. Berkeley: University of California Press.

Zarowsky, C., Haddad, S., & Nguyen, V.-K. (2013). Beyond "vulnerable groups": Contexts and dynamics of vulnerability. *Global Health Promotion, 20*(1 suppl.), 3–9.

Zientek, D., & Bonnell, R. (2020). When international humanitarian or medical missions go wrong: An ethical analysis. *HEC Forum, 32*(4), 333–343. https://doi.org/10.1007/s10730-019-09392-6.

# INDEX

Abimbola, Seye, 123
access to care, 115–16
accountability: DIY global health and, 8; jornada care and, 96; lack of, 117–24; visceral ethics and, 126
Adams, Vincanne, 9, 19
Addiss, David, 119
affect, 4, 138n4; development industry and, 138n6; ethics and, 63; global health and, 113–17, 132; visceral ethics and, 126
affordability, 129
albendazole, 39–40
Ali, Daud, 10–11
Amon, Joseph, 119
anencephaly, 105
anthelmintics, 39–40, 144n27
anthropology: gift giving analyses in, 72; global health and, 5–6; humanitarianism and, 9; place and, 18; virtue ethics and, 6
anti-Indigenous racism, 126
antiretroviral therapies (ARVs), 19
Aristotle, 79, 139n13
ARVs. *See* antiretroviral therapies
austerity measures, 28–29, 142n10

Bauman, Zygmunt, 6
Behrhorst, Carroll, 141n2
Behrhorst clinic, 25, 28, 141n2
best practices, 140n20
Biehl, João, 5, 139n16
bioethics, 64; privacy and, 146n1
biomedical interventions, 87; influence of wider structures and, 106
Birn, Anne-Emanuelle, 39

Biruk, Cal, x, 137n2
Black Lives Matter, 126
body knowledge, 16, 63–64; ethical action and, 76
Bornstein, Erica, 9, 70, 141n3
Brada, Betsey, 10, 147n6
Brocher Declaration, 128–29, 152n17
Brock, Karen, 44
Brown, Theodore, 28

cardiac surgery, 114–15
cascade iatrogenesis, 117
cervical cancer, xiv, 108
Chary, Anita, 117–18
Child Survival campaign, 27
choice-focused narrative, 107
Christian medical missionaries, 26, 143n15
citizen aid, 144n26
Citrin, David, 77
civic engagement, 46
clinical global health travel, 46
clothing, 137n4
Cold War, 142n7
Cole, Teju, 127
colonial ways of thinking, 122–23
colonization: "civilizing mission" of, 33; DIY global health and, 123; global health and, 63; international health and, 31–32; medical missions and, 32–33, 38; quinine and, 33; STMMs and, 33; tropical medicine and, 26
communication skills, 99
community health worker programs, 141n2

173

## ABOUT THE AUTHOR

NICOLE S. BERRY is Professor in the Faculty of Health Sciences at Simon Fraser University and the author of *Unsafe Motherhood: Mayan Maternal Mortality and Subjectivity in Post-war Guatemala.*